BIKE SMART

THINGS EVERY BICYCLIST SHOULD KNOW

WRITTEN AND ILLUSTRATED

BY

RUDOLPH J. POYORENA

All rights reserved.

First copyright © 2023 by RUDOLPH J. POYORENA

978-1-945677-98-4

No part of this book may be reproduced or transmitted in any form or by any means, electronic or mechanical, including photocopying, recording, or by any information storage and retrieval system, without the permission of the author.

Notice

This book/ebook is designed to provide motivation and information to its readers. The author assumes no responsibility for any personal injury, property damage, or any loss of any sort suffered from any actions taken based on or inspired by the information or advice presented in this book. Make sure you completely understand any procedure before beginning work. If in doubt, consult or get help from a competent mechanic. If you choose to apply the ideas in this book/ebook, you take full responsibility for your actions.

INTRODUCTION

The humble bicycle has been around for a long time. Since its inception, it has been a wonderful, romantic way to discover one's freedom and find adventure—truly a tool to indulge the senses and spirit of exploration.

Here we have a two-wheeled device to wander where few powered vehicles can, like the narrow-trailed byways and the roads less traveled, those scenic routes whose boundaries are only limited by the power of a person to pedal.

It is also, and has been, a trusty workhorse to go from point A to point B, and to get a person to his/her job without needing a drop of gas. This makes it incredibly attractive as a mode of transportation for saving money, giving freedom from pump dependency and allowing a person to become greener. Not to mention its appeal in being relatively simple, low maintenance and unanimously fun. In this modern age of advancements, the bicycle has truly become quite a practical and magnificent machine.

This sporty marvel has taken on a great many different varieties, unlike that of its predecessors long ago with only a few main styles to choose from. Now, there are specific bicycles available for every purpose under the sun. All meticulously engineered and made to suit for its own purpose.

Simply put, there is not just one bicycle that does it all, for all applications. For that reason, many types continue to be developed as more needs arise.

That being said, the bicycle has not really changed all that much since the creation of the "Rover Safety Bicycle" by John Kemp Starley, debuting in 1885. This design set the pattern for the modern bicycle: two wheels, pneumatic tires, a diamond frame, saddle, handlebars and chain drive. Yes, it has been improved through the years by using different frame geometries, lighter and stronger materials, computer assisted designs, better gearing, shocks, and modern fabricating techniques, but all in all, it's basically the same.

And since all bikes are similar, it stands to reason that the needs of every rider everywhere would be similar too. I find this to be unanimously true and undeniably evident. And upon considering this, the question arises, "What does a bicyclist need most?" To this I'd say, "The need for knowledge, no doubt." Yes, the absolute "musts" of riding in general, which are the essentials. For without those, a rider goes his/her way unprepared and at the mercy of his/her own ignorance. And since these bicycling "musts" cover much ground, they obviously would require a book to address them. Thus, I've written this book! I can epitomize these "musts" in a few words simply as a subtitle, as "**Things every bicyclist should know.**" My goal in this book is to focus on these common things. A person needs to have a good general understanding of his/her bicycle, along with knowledge of parts and basic repair. He/She needs to understand accessories and what to bring along for the ride. Also, what to wear, and other things that will make him/her a better and more proficient rider, a smarter rider!

In my book, *BIKE SMART: THINGS EVERY BICYCLIST SHOULD KNOW*, I will share what I have learned over many years of riding, having ridden various kinds of these brilliant machines. This is not a repair manual. It's a book to convey very practical and common-sense information and tips that will help you save time, money and needless hardships as you venture into the streets and backways to explore your bliss or go to work. Remember that a well-equipped and knowledgeable rider not only helps himself, but also riders who may need assistance on the road. I am confident that after carefully reading this book, you will feel more able to do both.

TABLE OF CONTENTS

CHAPTERS

1) BIKE SMART - THE ART OF CHOOSING YOUR RIDE

2) PREP SMART - THE ART OF PREPPING YOUR NEW BIKE

3) PART SMART - THE ART OF THE GAME CHANGER PARTS

4) ACCESSORY SMART - THE ART OF CHOOSING ACCESSORIES

5) PACK SMART - THE ART OF WHAT TO BRING

6) GEAR SMART - THE ART OF WHAT TO WEAR

7) RIDE SMART - THE ART OF THE SAFE RIDE

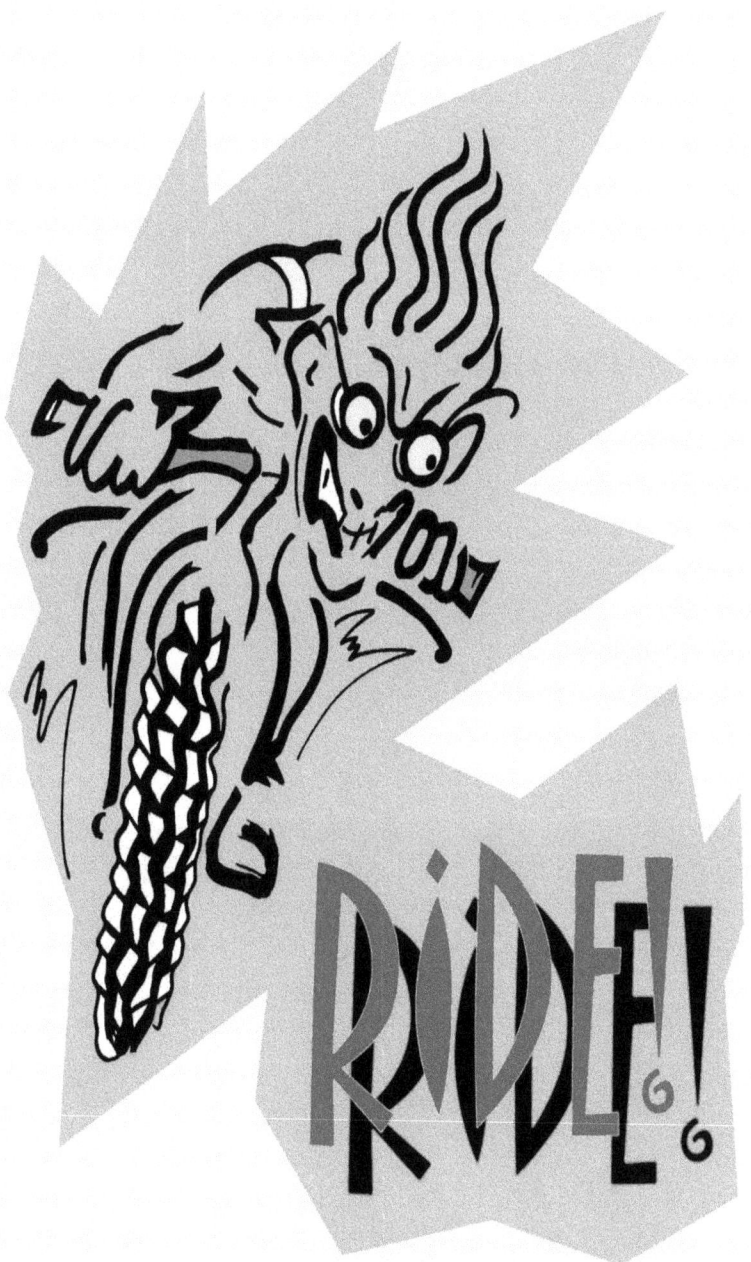

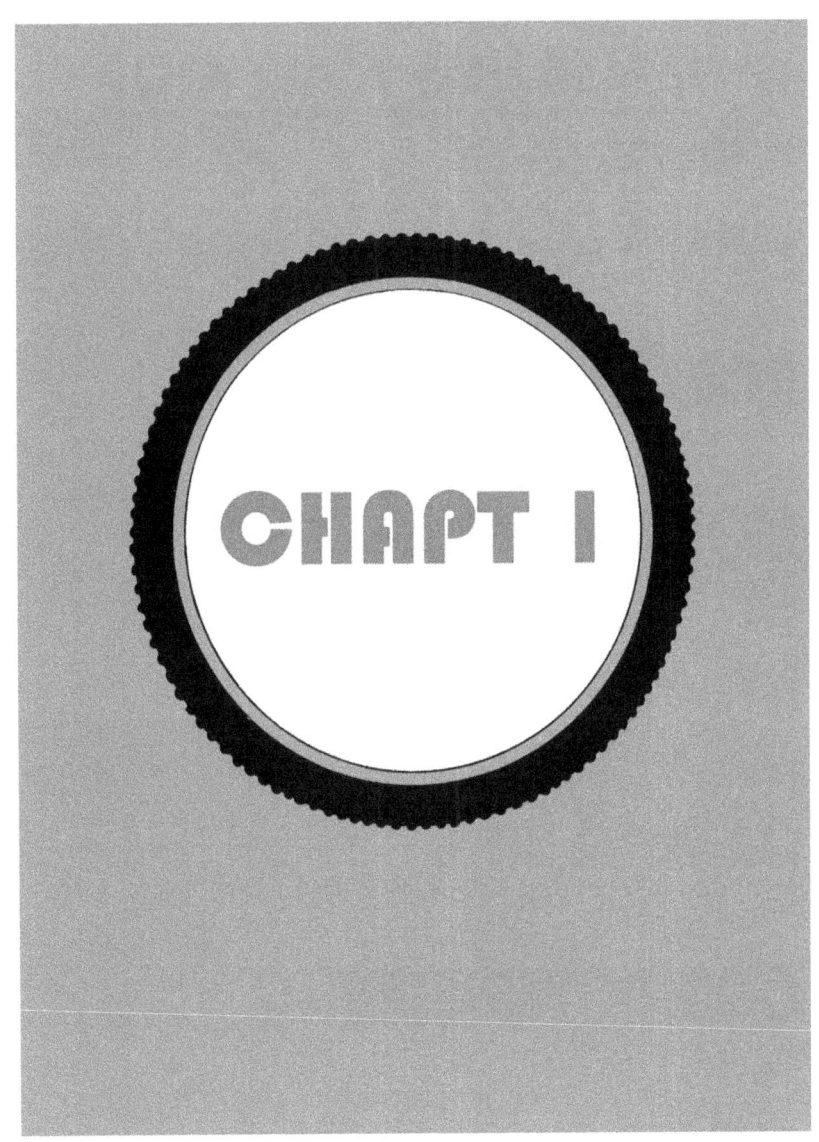

BIKE SMART - THE ART OF CHOOSING YOUR RIDE

WHERE DO I START?

ROAD BIKE

MOUNTAIN BIKE

HYBRID BIKE

CRUISER BIKE

COMMUTER BIKE

FIXIE

GRAVEL BIKE THE NITTY-GRITTY OF THE PURCHASE

WHERE DO I START?

KEEPING IT SIMPLE!

YOU NEED SOME WHEELS! What kind? Where do I go to buy some? Hold on! To properly weigh out the task of getting your ride, you need some basic information presented in a logical sequence. And, in order to understand anything complicated (the bike being one), you also need to break it down to its most understandable elements. Let me begin...

Choosing a bike these days is not as simple as deciding on a road bike, mountain bike or cruiser bike? There are many more varieties of "bike types" available. And beyond these "bike types," there are also additional "variations" or "offshoots" to these "bike types." So, these days it's more like, what kind of road bike and what kind of mountain bike? And what about hybrids, where do they fit in? This makes a simple selection more complicated and mind-spinning. Yes, choices upon choices! But you must start somewhere. And for starters, you must go back to basic "bike type." So, to break it down, I'll stick to the first two most basic bike-buying deliberations, which are "bike type" and "cost." That's a good place to start!

"BIKE TYPE" & "COST"

Having a good idea of what "type of bike" one needs and "what one is willing to spend" are foremost and always the place to begin in a bike purchase. Only when these two factors are decided upon can one later move on to the finer details of "variation of a type," its options, and size, as considerations. If this is not self-explanatory enough, I'll explain it further in a different way. Think of it like this. The "bike type" represents a path to go (what type and where to find this type of bike!). And "what one is willing to spend" represents a means, and its limits (here's my bottom line!). Put them together and presto! You have a clear starting point. "Variation" (what version?) is contemplated further down the road. Makes sense! And now, you need to consider your path as to "bike type." I'll talk about money later.

NOTE: "Types" of bikes vary greatly in price. For example, a sport road bike will cost more than a basic mountain bike. So, a person's choice in "type" can be dictated by the wallet alone. Something to think about!

DIRECTION

Given here is an overview on common "bike types" and uses. I will go into further detail about them and their specifics and pros and cons later in this chapter. But for now, you need a path. Knowing what exists and their uses will help to steer you and make you aware of general "bike types," and further on down their "variations." So, logically, this primer is needed to dip your feet. Here is a brief on types of bikes to help you. Let us explore...

NOTE: I do consider hybrid bikes, comfort bikes, commuter bikes, fixies and gravel bikes as "bike types" and not "variations."

BASIC BIKES

THE ROAD BIKE: These bikes are mostly for sport and speed, and some are made for trekking long distances. These are strictly for smooth roads because their tires are narrow, but some can be furnished with wider tires for harsher roads. Most road bikes can also be outfitted for commuter use, but "racing types" are not ideal for that purpose, because their aggressive ride position favors speed and not overall traffic visuals.

THE MOUNTAIN BIKE: 26-, 27.5- or 29-inch (wheel size) "hard-tail" (front shock only) mountain bikes are good for most road and terrain uses. They are good multi-purpose bikes, even for commuting medium distances.

THE HYBRID BIKE: These bikes are a cross between a road bike and mountain bike. They are particularly good for fitness, commuting, and light gravel roads, as there are different versions. They can also be outfitted for various uses, including trekking and commuting. They are very versatile, light, and fast. Most hybrids have an upright riding position and are favorable for commuting.

THE CRUISER BIKE: These are good bikes for short leisure rides and are extremely comfortable. Single-speed bikes are not suited for long distances, but their low maintenance and comfort are their charm.

THE COMMUTER BIKE: These bikes are suited for city purposes. They usually have moustache, or riser bars, fenders, and a rear rack.

THE FIXIE: These minimalist, single-speed bikes are for flat city riding.

THE GRAVEL BIKE: This is the new kid on the block as far as bikes are concerned. They may look like a road bike, but are specifically designed and geared for light off-road and gravel applications.

SIMPLE! THE "BIKE TYPE" YOU WILL NEED TO BUY IS DECIDED BY ITS PURPOSE.

CONSIDER THESE THINGS

Now that you are getting your feet wet, you have a general idea of the bike categories that are out there. You can now begin to narrow down "bike type" by YOUR PURPOSE; later you can scrutinize "variation" and "details." Thinking about these things below will add some clarity to the process.

1) If your bike is going to be used for exercise or sport:

Then you can start looking into road and hybrid bikes as a "bike type." "Variation," gearing, and weight are things to further consider.

2) If your bike is only going to be used for commuting:

Then you can start looking into hybrid and commuter bikes as a "bike type." "Variation" and needed rack mounts on the frame are things to be further considered.

3) If your bike is only going to be used for trips to the store:

Then you can start looking into cruiser, commuter, entry level mountain and hybrid bikes as a "bike type." Theft protection, accessories, and needed rack mounts on the frame are things to be further considered. Contemplate also whether you are going to leave your bike unattended for long periods of time.

4) If your bike is primarily going to be used for long distance commuting:

Then you can start looking into road (general) and hybrid bikes as a "bike type." "Variation," rider position, tire tread, wheel size, needed rack mounts on the frame, and weight are things to be further considered.

5) If your bike is going to be used for both gravel and hills:

Then you can start looking into an entry level mountain, gravel or all-terrain hybrid bike (being a variation of hybrid bike) as a "bike type." Suspension and tire width need to be further considered.

   Yes, there are lots of things to think about in choosing a bike (assuming you are somewhat familiar with the terms above). And many things must be thought out in advance. The details count. So, it is prudent to go into your choice and further purchase with as much information as you can. I will try to fill in the blanks.

GOT AN INKLING?

HERE IS THAT SECOND

FACTOR TO CONSIDER:

COST!

Your budget: This **DETERMINES** where you are going to buy your new bike, bike store or department store? Online or yard sale? It also influences your **CHOICES** as I said. So, you might want to keep saving your money to broaden your selection so that you are not limited. Besides the price of a bike, there are many extra items needed for cycling that will increase the amount of green stuff needed. I will get into these items later in this book.

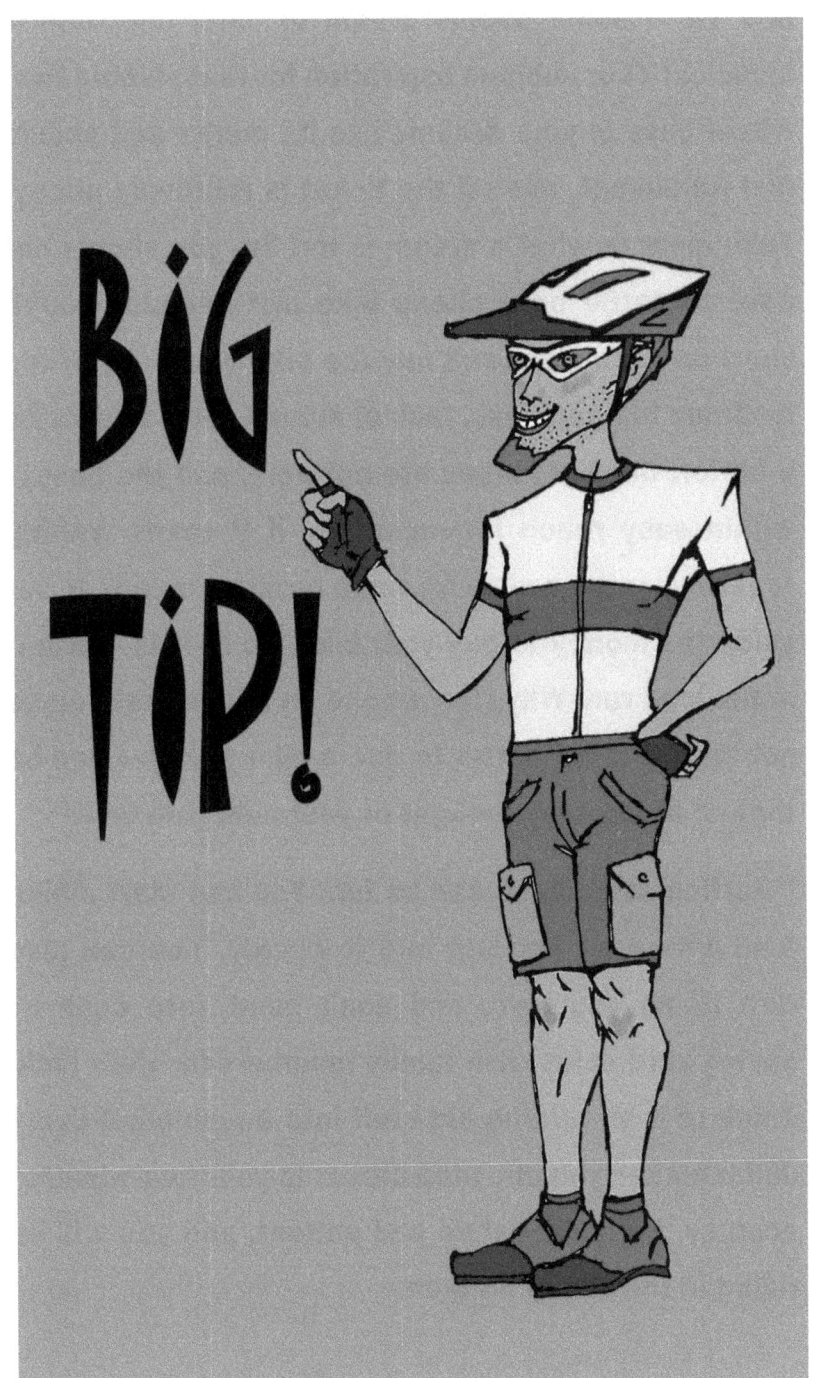

BIG TIP – Some people dream of cars, and others, bicycles! Your sublime aspiration for that shining two-wheel bliss of your dreams has its merits and should find fulfillment, even if the ticket is relatively pricey. Fulfillment is what a dream is for! So, you should not have to settle on a cheap bike just because you're short on cash and can't buy the bike you want. When it comes to happiness, lack of money should never be a factor. Besides, bikes are not cars, and the cost is within easy reach for most. So, if it takes waiting several months and using some creative means to set aside the money to buy your bike, do it! It is worth it in the long run. Why ride around on a bike that you do not like? It is far better to ride a bike you love and be thrilled at the very thought of your next ride on it!

Setting aside cash can be fun. You can start a bike fund with a jar and put into it weekly. You can also turn items you own, and don't need, into cash by having yard sales. Ask family members for their junk. Think of it as turning old stuff into a new bike! Every dollar makes you one step closer to your two-wheeled ecstasy. So, be creative and patient, and you will be riding in the sun in no time.

YOU HAVE AN IDEA OF WHAT YOU NEED, BUT STILL UNSURE? OK, LET'S NOW DIG DEEPER INTO THE PARTICULARS OF GENERAL "BIKE TYPES" AND THEIR "VARIATIONS"

Here again are the general types of bikes, as lightly discussed earlier, but now in detail. Here I will go into their functions, limitations, and pros and cons. After reading, you can make a confident and conclusive determination of a "bike type."

ROAD BIKE

"Road bikes" are very specific bikes. They are built for speed and sport. They are restricted to the paved road, except for "gravel bikes," which have become a new "bike type" rather than just a "variation" of road bike. Their curled handlebars (drop bars) are made for three riding positions. They are lightweight and geared to ride fast and far. There are many "variations" of road bikes, and the choices abound.

To the untrained eye, all road bikes appear pretty much the same, except for the noticeable graphics. But the nuances are many. Some road bike "variations," such as touring bikes, are built for long distance traveling. They can be outfitted with panniers and racks because they come with rack mounts. Their geometry is worked out for comfort and less road fatigue. For example, they usually have a fork that is noticeably curved forward to reduce shock, unlike the sport type which has a straight fork.

Others are middle ground road bikes and have a broader range of use, so their features are universal to road bikes. And still others are specifically designed for racing, as their low stem height and frame geometry encourages a racing position.

Among the various road bikes, many have different types of shifting mechanisms. And these different types of shifters can considerably add or subtract from the cost of the bike. Also, many have different places where these shifters are mounted. This can be a major issue whose ramifications are not fully apparent until after one buys and rides the bike. Such is the case of shifters mounted to the down tube. So, be aware!

The road bike frame has changed the least over the years. The same can be said of old commuter bikes with moustache bars, which is essentially a road bike with upright bars.

The pros to this class of bike are: light, fast, sporty, tight in braking, and the gold standard for long distances. Cons are: limited to smooth road riding (excluding gravel bikes), hunched rider position and a jolty ride depending on the quality of road.

TIP – Consider well the area in which you live and the condition of the streets and paving. A road bike is limited, and a limited bike has narrow practicality.

NOTE: I find road bikes that have their shifters located on the down tube to be unsafe and awkward at best, because in the action of making a gear shift, a rider:

- Is forced to take one hand off the handlebar.
- Takes his/her eyes off the road to locate the shifter.
- Reaches down to shift the shifter (stability issue).

All these motions have a potential to cause accidents. And considering the many times gear shifts are made in traffic situations, one can clearly see a shifter such as this is not practical. This is a classic feature used in older racing bikes that is still used today. It does have a bottom-line value because it saves the manufacturers money by them not having to furnish their bikes with expensive two-fold brake/shifter mechanism combos. All that's required here are two simple hand brakes and two shift levers. So, this is super minimalist as far as shifter mechanisms are concerned. I feel this feature should be relegated to the past and dismissed as old technology, or at best, used only for true racing applications. But, for the purposes of the average cyclist, shifters should be located on, or as close to, the handlebars as possible. This is safer and less cumbersome.

MOUNTAIN BIKE

There are many "variations" of "Mountain bikes." There is downhill, trail, big drop, cross-country, and cross-trails, to name a few. Mountain bikes in general share a frame geometry that offers much desired room between the rider and top tube, unlike that of most road bikes. This is accomplished by its frame being constructed with a sloping top tube. Also, the frames are thick, compact and designed to be strong. These bikes are built to tackle rough terrain and geared for going uphill. They have fat knobby tires, a front shock (entry level bike), and riser bars. Because it goes outside the scope of this book, which is general cycling. I'll stick to "hardtail" (front shock only) mountain bikes, which are all-purpose and not specific to the hardcore sport.

Mountain bikes these days have different wheel sizes to choose from. This is a big consideration that affects your riding, and likely which bike you ultimately choose, so it's worth discussing. When mountain bikes first began, they started out with 26-inch wheels. Back in the day that was all they had as far as rough terrain wheels are concerned, so they used what they had. Now there are 27.5-inch and 29-inch wheel sizes.

29-inch wheels, also known as 29ers, make quick work of the hills, with the least amount of effort, flowing/rolling properties, and big bike feel. You just simply roll over everything. But due to this large wheel size, the rider does seem to lose some sense of connection between the bike and the ground. Also, a strange phenomenon associated with them is that they have a slow-motion effect on the downhill. I can attest to this.

The 26-inch wheels, on the other hand, are strong, proven wheels, but their size is outdated and seems ridiculously small after riding bigger wheels. They are definitely on their way out, and rightly so.

The 27.5-inch wheel is a happy medium and is the sweet spot in concerns with wheel size. This size is the modern standard now.

Besides the overall size of wheel, there is also tire width to consider. For example, a 26x2-inch knobby tire is best suited for mountain riding and a bit too bulky for the road. But a thinner (and not much) 26x1.95-inch knobby is good for all road, gravel, and small hill applications; but, not really suited for real mountain biking. So, small variations of width will change riding dynamics. Beyond width, there is also tire tread pattern to further ponder.

A mountain bike gives a lot of room as far as modifying your ride. Modifying your bike can add new life to your bike and change its overall feel drastically. It's a given that you are going to alter some things on a mountain bike, whether out of the shop or in the shop. Customizing is typical. Upgrading or changing out your stem, handlebars, grips or tires will enhance your bike and make it feel totally different and better (I will go into further detail later, in Chapter 3).

More to consider: Front shock or rigid fork? Some mountain bikes come with a front shock; some come with a rigid fork. The suspension fork or front shock on a hardtail mountain bike offers comfort on the trail and road. It gives a cushy ride. But it does steal a little momentum from the down stroke in hard pedaling, slowing you down a bit. This is more noticeable on flat, long-distance road rides. Whereas, with rigid forks, no energy is lost, but you get a harder ride. So, suspension shock or rigid fork? This needs to be considered.

A cool variation of the mountain bike is the single-speed mountain bike. These are either sold as single-speed or are a normal mountain bike modified to be a single-speed via conversion kit. A single-speed mountain bike can have a front shock or rigid fork. These are coveted bikes because of their minimalist nature, which is liberating and carefree! But you will either love them or hate them. No shifters, no derailleurs, minimal maintenance, lighter weight and fewer cables, what's not to love? Single speed means you work harder, especially on the incline. And on the long roads you'll be spinning your cranks to little avail, lacking the gears that make you fast. So, you might hate them going up a hill or on a straightaway. But in the process of working harder, they make you a better rider and strengthen your legs more than a geared bike.

Single-speed mountain bikes have different gearing ratios. That means they use varying combinations of chainring and cog sizes for different riding applications. These sizes equate to number of teeth on each chainring and cog. The first number is chainring teeth and the second is cog teeth. On a 26-inch bike, for example, some ratios or number of teeth can be 42:17 or 40:17 for road riding, 39:18 for trail riding, and 32:17 for hill riding. There is the so-called "divine gearing," a gearing that works well with almost all riding. The "divine gearing" is 34:21. These ratios are examples, because they may not exactly translate the same for different wheel sizes and may give a different riding result. Remember, all ratios are built on personal preference to begin with. There is no exact ratio, only what works best for each individual rider. Yes, a single-speed can be a very tailored ride!

All in all, mountain bikes are the most versatile and multi-purpose bikes, lending themselves to a gambit of personal touches and accessory additions. The mountain bike has proven itself as strong and dependable. These bikes, if maintained well, can last a great many years. They say the life expectancy of a bike is about five years. That's nonsense. This would be true only if you leave it to the elements, don't do regular maintenance, or just ride it to the ground. A well-made bike can last decades. So, in choosing a bike, a mountain bike should be high up there on the list for most riding purposes and bike longevity.

The pros to this class of bike are: versatility, strength, modification friendly, a forgiving ride, and no fear of the road or trail hindrances.

Cons are: some very minimal loss of momentum due to a suspension fork, and due to the small wheel circumference, 26-inch wheel size mountain bikes are no good for long distances.

TIP – Consider that a wide application bike, such as a mountain bike, is a useful and reliable form of transportation in an emergency, given its ability to cover all terrains. Outfitted with racks, panniers, cages, and water bottles, this bike would be considered an ideal bug out vehicle in a disaster or crisis situation. In addition, having a bike cargo trailer would greatly add to the load carrying capacity of your bike, if bugging out was for an extended length of time. These can be bought ready for use or improvised from an old two-wheeled bike child carrier. A mountain bike is the best bike to consider for emergency purposes off and on the trail.

NOTE 1: The 26-inch wheel size mountain bike has been a universal mainstay as far as mountain bikes are concerned. It has always been easy to obtain tires, tubes, and wheels, due to the abundance of their availability. But that is apparently coming to an end, as I said. Bike shops have now phased them out in favor of the 27.5-inch wheel size (except for certain small rider and female bikes). The 26-inch wheel mountain bike is mostly available now in department stores and online, and in mostly cheap versions.

The 27.5-inch new modern standard, in my opinion, is even more universal in application than the 26-inch wheel, and can even handle long distance rides with no problem. I find that even their 2-inch width tires are not an issue of weight or sluggishness. I have only good things to say about this wheel size, and I definitely would not go back to 26-inch wheels.

NOTE 2: Remember that 24-inch wheels and below are not for adults. These are kid sizes, and an adult will look foolish if they insist on riding a bike with small wheels. The only two exceptions are (1) if an adult is very, very short, or (2) the folding mini type bikes for adults, made to be compact and adjustable for any size person.

NOTE 3: To find the size of any wheel, simply look at the side of the tire.

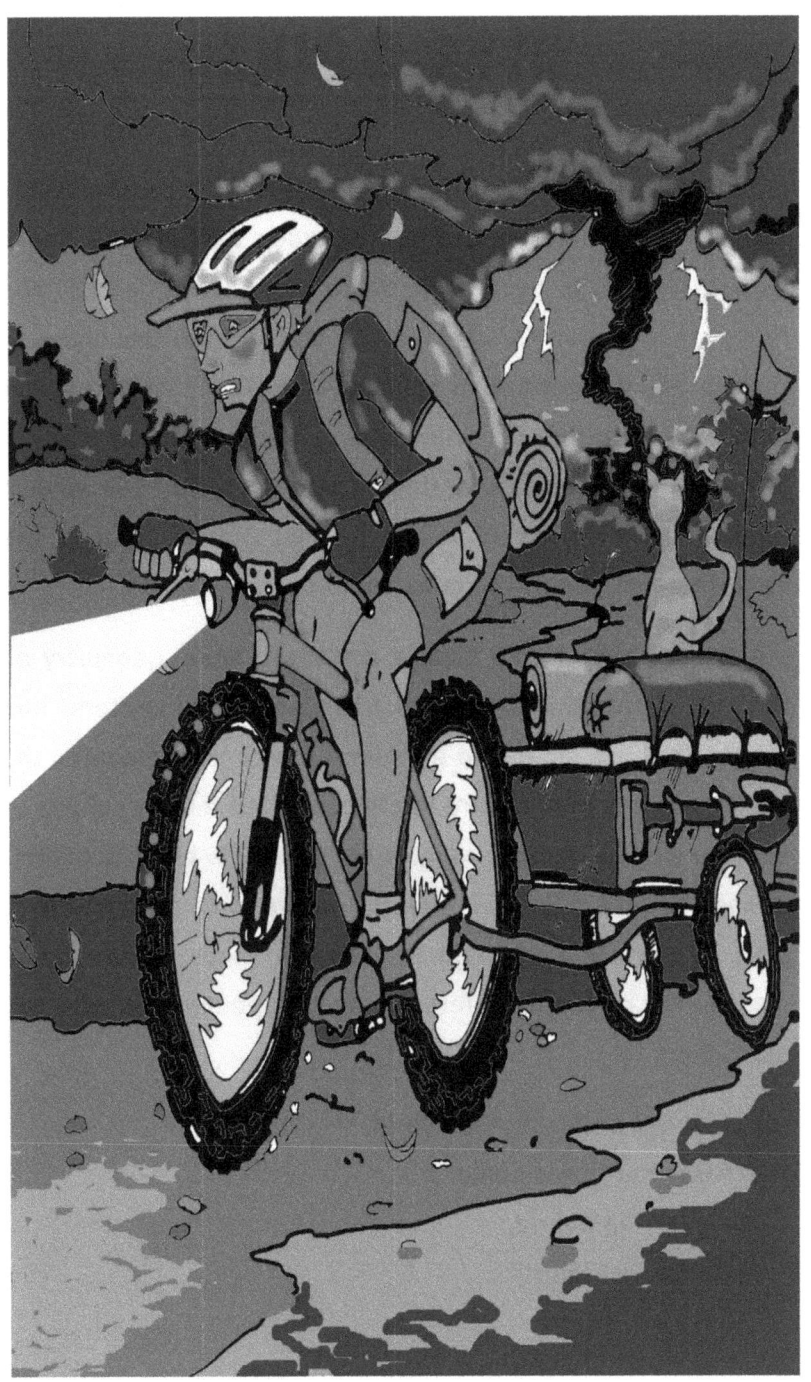

HYBRID BIKE

The "Hybrid bike" is a cross between a road bike and a mountain bike, in general. It has a great many merits, and there are also many kinds of hybrid offshoots to this class. In reality, this classification spills over to kinds of bikes that have existed before the name was coined, as well as many in between bikes that are springing up today. So, it is kind of hard to get a fix on what a hybrid is. But I'll stick to the definition and general form as we know it today.

A typical hybrid bike shares the same basic geometry as that of a mountain bike, and has riser bars, shifters, and brakes that are similar to a mountain bike. But it shares the wheel size and general tire thickness (often thicker) of a road bike, as well as its light weight. These nimble bikes also offer a more upright riding position not afforded to a typical road bike. There are four major classes of these bikes. These classes are called by different names depending on who you are talking to:

1) Flat bar performance hybrid.
2) Riser bar fitness bike.
3) All-terrain hybrid.
4) Commuter hybrid.

The "Flat bar performance hybrid" is similar to a road bike in most respects. In fact, the only difference from it being an actual road bike are its handlebars, shifters, and brakes.

The "Riser bar fitness bike," is middle ground between the "flat bar performance hybrid" and the "all-terrain hybrid." This bike's frame geometry has more in common with a mountain bike, but it is a true road bike in its intention. When people think of a hybrid bike, this model usually comes to mind, because it is the midpoint between road and mountain bike.

The "All-terrain hybrid" looks like a mountain bike, with its rugged frame and a front shock. The only discernable difference from that of a mountain bike is its thinner width hybrid 700c tire size.

And lastly, the "Commuter hybrid," which is an enigma. This bike may have an appearance that is typically hybrid, but it also has a look that is not categorical. It can have 26-inch wheels with a suspension fork, or 700c wheels with a rigid fork. It can also look similar to a traditional city bike, with fenders and rack, and have varying handlebar types. So, as to where a commuter hybrid ends, and a commuter bike begins, that is up for debate.

Hybrids are great bikes for long distances, errands, short trips, and general fitness workouts. Their 700c wheels roll with ease and cover large distances effortlessly. They are also very agile. And after riding a mountain bike for years, I can clearly appreciate the virtues of this kind of bike. There is so much positive to say about these bikes and hardly anything negative, other than the unyielding nature of the straight fork on those bikes, causing a hard ride. But a change to wider tires is the usual remedy. By and large, this is another bike that should be up there on the list.

Pros to this class of bike are: upright riding position, rolling ease, nimble, light, modification friendly, and excellent for long distances.

The Con is that the straight fork on non-suspension models makes for a hard ride on bad roads.

TIP – Since hybrids are primarily road bikes (excluding the "all-terrain hybrid"), you may still be able to boost the functionality by adding fatter tires. Most hybrids come with a 700x32c tire, which is a road only tire. But by upgrading to a 700x38c tire and wider (see note below), you can add light gravel roads to your bike's uses.

NOTE 1: In choosing a hybrid bike, make sure the fork and frame have the option for fatter tires. This most likely would not be the case of a flat bar performance hybrid, but very likely on all other variations. The choice of a hybrid tire is limited to the inner width of the fork, seatstay, and chainstay, as all bikes are. So, if you are planning to change out your tires to larger width tires, make sure your hybrid fork and frame can accommodate these.

NOTE 2: Before you try to beef up your hybrid, consider this: a hybrid is a mixture of road bike and mountain bike by design.

Its leaning is to rougher road riding beyond what a road bike can handle. It is proudly a middle ground bike and makes no claim to being a mountain bike. Even the "all-terrain hybrid" has its limitations, simply because it is not a true mountain bike. Its tire width and frame are not built for all-out mountain riding. Light trails and gravel roads are where it shines. So, trying to turn a hybrid into a mountain bike will not work. You might as well just go all the way and buy a 29er mountain bike, which would be its wheel size equivalent. That being said, there's nothing wrong with upping the tire size on a hybrid, provided you ride it like a hybrid.

CRUISER BIKE

The "Cruiser bike" is a simple yet stylish bike used for cruising the beach. Often colorful, and classic looking, cruisers usually have large upright chrome handlebars that allow a relaxed position while riding. The geometry is such that the riding position is as though one is sitting while riding. They come with a large, cushioned seat and fat white-walled tires. Most of these only have one speed and fenders.

The older cruisers, as well as most of the newer ones, have a one-piece crank that is trouble-free. This one-piece crank has been around for a long time. In fact, not much has changed in the basic overall design of these bikes, and the retro look is always in vogue. They maintain a classy look and give a fun and uncomplicated ride.

An off-road variation of cruiser bike is what is called a "Klunker bike." A "Klunker bike" is a single-speed cruiser bike dressed in dirt bike handlebars, BMX stem, knobby tires and a road bike saddle. This is essentially the first mountain bike, and is old school bike riding at best. People convert old beach cruisers into klunkers. But they especially seek out the old heavy-duty cruisers that have a double-curve top tube, which can take more abuse. A klunker is versatile, rugged, and pure fun. The two best things about a klunker are you don't have to dress-up to ride and the more weathered they get, the better they look.

A "Comfort bike," which is a kind of cruiser bike, has become a new class (type) of bike. These bikes allow for an even more relaxed sitting position than a classic cruiser by having a lower seat geometry and crank positioning that is more forward. These come in single-speed and in multi-speed versions. Their handlebars are usually a 3-to-4-inch riser bar, not a classic cruiser bar. And the saddle is more of a comfort commuter bike saddle.

Pros of a classic cruiser bike are: sturdy, simple, fun, relaxed riding position, and most have bolted wheels that are better for bike security.

Cons are: heavy, need a wrench for flat fixing. And as far as classic cruisers are concerned, wide handlebars make for tight riding in traffic. These bikes are not good for, nor made for, uphill use or long distances.

Pros of comfort bikes are: fun, relaxed riding position and they bring back the pleasure of the simple ride.

The con is that even the geared versions will not ascend uphill easily, due to the rider position.

NOTE: Cruiser and comfort bikes are great for flat road riding and feeling the good vibrations along the beach trails.

COMMUTER BIKE

A "Commuter bike" is pretty much any bike that is set aside for the purpose of going to work, school or the supermarket. That being said, most bikes that are specifically made for commuting have upright moustache handlebars and a cushy saddle. So, there is a specific image in mind when the words "commuter bike" comes up. There are exceptions to this image, given the rise of modern urban commuter bikes, a newer category to an older type of bike, which look more contemporary. "Commuter bikes" usually have fenders and a medium tire thickness leaning towards the thin side. They can have a back rack and the usual accessories needed for city riding.

In many countries and cities in Europe, especially Amsterdam and the country of Denmark, archaic commuter bikes serve to get people to work and are a big part of the social way of transportation. Commuter bikes are everywhere and used for most everything. They have a bicycle culture, and riding a bike is not even remotely considered a poor man's transport; it is the norm. This bicycle culture promotes the idea of being green, and it is cool too! Small families can be seen on multifunctional cargo bikes that have large "compartment areas" in front of the bike for the children. These "compartment areas" double for carrying groceries as well. The streets are very bicycle-friendly and oriented. Here in America, we are beginning to see the value of commuting on bike as modeled by these countries. And as a result, cities are modifying streets to accommodate cyclists by painting bike lanes. Old or new, the highly functional commuter bike is paving its way from the past into the future.

All in all, a commuter bike is a pleasure workhorse. It may not be the prettiest bike in the garage, given its job, so you don't have to dress up to ride on this one either. There are really no pros or cons to this class of bike. It is what it is. It can be a mix of many bikes put together made to serve and carry, or purchased new for the task. In reality, any bike can be modified to be a commuter style bike. It's actually a fun project and a more personal ride. It is both leisure and work bike, and very likely, your favorite bike of all.

TIP – Moustache bars offer a super fun and extremely comfortable ride. Even though they are antiquated in style, they provide a riding position that allows the rider to see well in most directions, and are likely superior for overall observability. That is probably why they never went out of use in Europe. You can modernize the look of them by buying black colored ones, giving them a more fashionable avant-garde look. Also, plastic fenders have a real purpose, keeping watery street muck off you. So, embrace both of them. I do fully understand that most riders identify with the style and the type of bicycle they ride. Still, it will not hurt to try something new, by trying something old. You might like it!

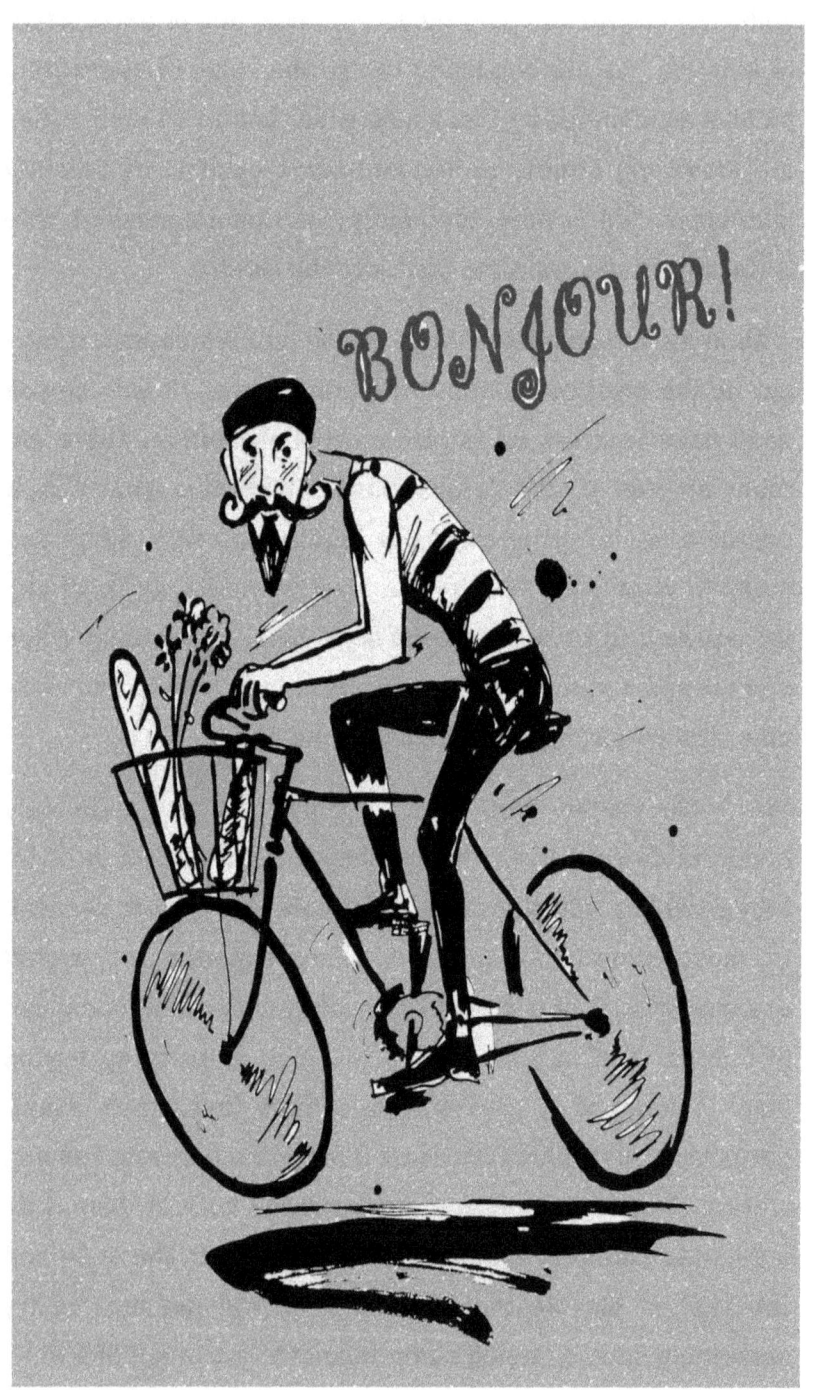

FIXIE

The "Fixie" is a simple ultra-minimalist bike. It is a steel framed, old-school bike stripped down to the very essentials and given a new hip look. It can have a narrow riser bar or flat bar, and usually has only one brake, and sometimes none! It is a single-speed bike, having a flip-flop rear wheel that gives you the option to ride with a single-speed freewheel or a fixed cog. A fixed cog will not allow you to coast along while pedaling. But instead, you must always be pedaling while the bike is in motion, like a track bike. The "fixie" is a trendy bike that is good for errands and cutting through traffic. It's not a bike for those who love the creature comforts of different speeds, accessories, and who are cycle tech freaks. Neither is it for those who see their bike as a tool for adventure, or who like to cover long distances. This bike is for the urban minimalist, those who want the least number of gadgets to mess with and least amount of maintenance. The "fixie" brings back a sense of being young and free.

There are really no pros or cons to this bike.

GRAVEL BIKE

A "Gravel bike" is more of a mountain bike, with drop bars and no suspension, than a road bike with fat tires. These bikes are crafted with tough, yet streamlined frames, semi-wide tires, and are geared for the rock-strewn trail. They are not true mountain bikes, nor are they true road bikes, as they are gravel bikes, and their geometry attests to that. In fact, they probably would not be classified as a kind of hybrid, either, but hold their own as a new bike "type." A gravel bike is fully comfortable on loose rocky trails and hilly semi-rough paths. A versatile bike, good for bike packing and long backwoods excursions, attracting a full mix of adventurous cycling enthusiasts.

The popularity of these bikes has skyrocketed and their following has steadily increased, and it's safe to say that they are here to stay.

There are no pros or cons to this bike in that they are very new to the scene.

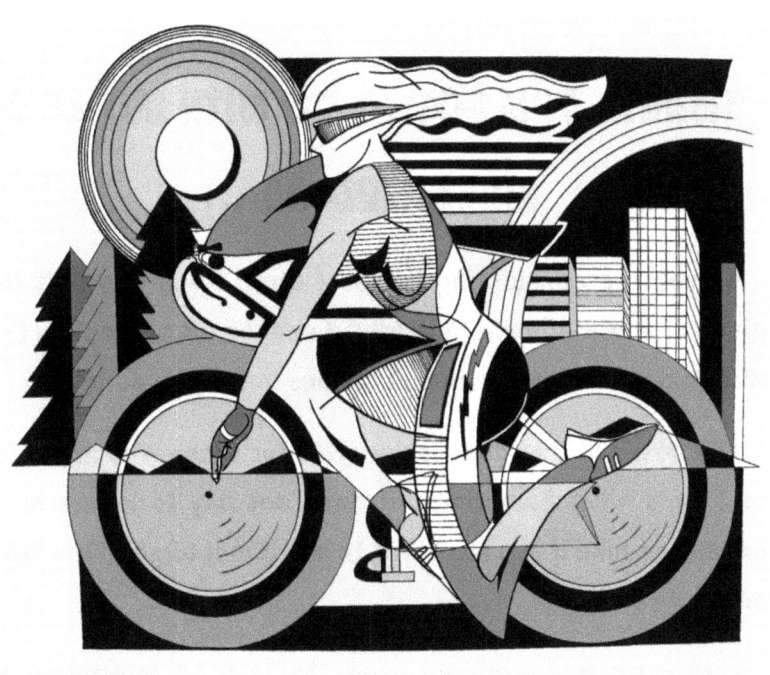

THEFT - I JUST LEFT IT FOR ONE MINUTE, NOW IT'S GONE!

(WHAT'S THIS GOT TO DO WITH BUYING A BIKE? READ ON...)

As you are considering loads of stuff, I will interject this piece of information here (oddly), because it's something that will no doubt influence any decisions you make early on.

The possibility of theft is very real for those who are going to own a bike. Sometimes it does not pay to invest in an expensive bike if you are going to use it just to go to the store or run errands.

Locks are not foolproof, and the best of locks can be opened. Further, a person with cable cutters can cut through a cable in a few seconds. So, it is best not to have a very tempting ride on display. An old bike may serve best for these purposes. Some people sticker and spray paint over a good bike to make it less appealing to thieves, which is a shame. Considering the possibility of theft, it would be suggested in this case to buy a department store bike or use an old bike (Read more in Chapter 7, **THEFT**).

YOU HAVE DECIDED ON THE "TYPE" AND "VARIATION" OF BIKE THAT BEST SUITS YOU, AND HAVE CASH IN POCKET, WHAT NOW?

THE NITTY-GRITTY OF THE PURCHASE

(AND MORE PARTICULARS)

BIKE STORE BIKE VS. DEPARTMENT STORE BIKE

Bike store bikes are always the way to go when purchasing a bike. Even the lowest end bikes in a bike store are more than sufficient in quality. These bikes are also built by trained and experienced bike mechanics and should be good-to-go out the door. Most bike stores also offer one free adjustment after your purchase. The price of a bike is sometimes negotiable, too. And keep in mind there are many sizes for a perfect fit, and usually two colors of the same bike to choose from. Sometimes tires and parts can be swapped out at the time of purchase for your more personalized preference. Also, you get the benefit of competent people to help guide you in your purchase and answer any questions you may have.

Department store bikes usually have good quality frames, but cheap components. Some of these department store bike frames are produced by the same large companies that make frames for bike store bikes. But the bars, shifters, derailleurs, seats, wheels, cranks, tires and bottom brackets are the cheapest they can source out to meet their bottom-line. The rims are usually single wall rims and are not as strong as bike store double wall rims. They usually have older type bottom brackets, too. Shifters are for the most part inexpensive twist grip (twist grip shifters suck, well, because they do). The handlebars are made of steel and are narrow. The components are often juggled in ways that present the bike in its best light. In other words, the cheapest parts are put in areas of the bike that are not noticed by your average consumer. Like the bottom bracket, for example.

As far as size is concerned, there are no custom fit sizes in department store bikes, there is just one size (medium) and color to choose from. This general size can be used by most riders of similar middle heights but are not optimal for a short or tall rider.

Also, they are supposed to be built (out of the box) by a competent bike builder, but if you look at them, it is easy to see they are not. I have noticed rows of bikes with forks put on backwards. Also, screws missing from stems. In addition, horribly positioned brake levers, handlebars, and shifters. There are a lot of upgrades that need to be made on these bikes to make them ride-worthy. So much so, you might as well buy a bike store bike to begin with. Department store bikes are meant to tantalize you with flashy colors and graphics to gloss over the fact that they are relatively cheap. Remember that the top-of-the-line department store bike is still below the bottom-of-the-line bike store bike. The only advantages to these bikes are the low price and the fact that the parts are usually under warranty with easy replacement.

A pet peeve of mine for department store bikes (and I have many) is the seatpost size. If you are a tall person and are going to buy a bike from a department store, check the length of the seatpost. Often, the bike will say that it is for tall riders, but the seatpost will not accommodate anyone above medium height. A tiny seatpost means you will have to purchase a longer one if you buy the bike. Also, the stems are usually too small.

NOTE: Buyer beware! A cheap mountain bike may have a suspension fork that shudders, sticks and makes popping and creaking sounds when in use. This can be very irritating on a ride. Even if you add lube, it will not help. It's just a cheap shock, and there's no fixing it. I know this firsthand. It's always better to have a rigid fork than a cheap creaky shock.

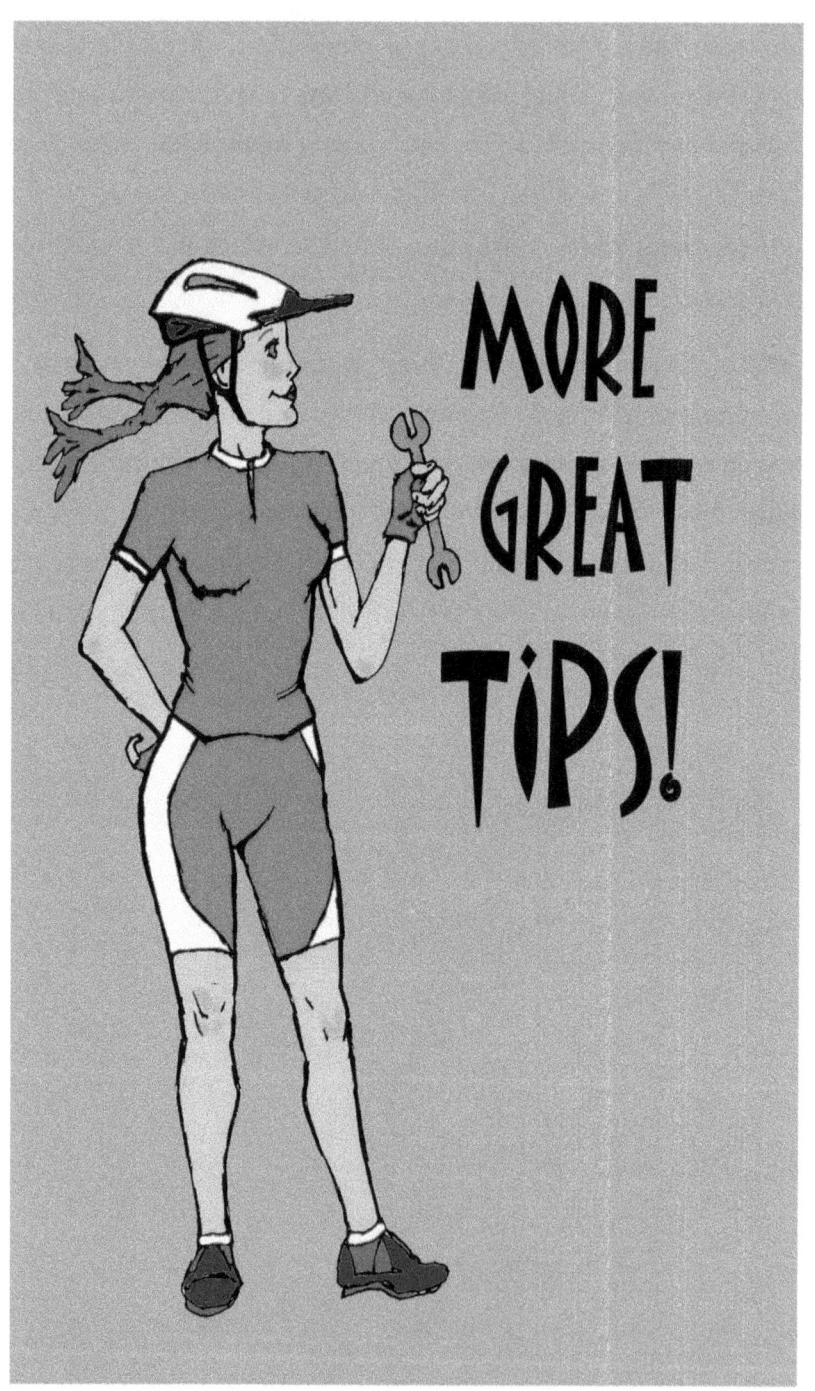

TIP 1 – Consider that sometimes a department store bike will have one wheel with a disc brake and another with a V-brake (which I find ridiculous).

TIP 2 – Department store bikes are notorious for having dry bearings. I guess they are produced so quickly that not much time is taken in greasing the bearings. It could also be the manufacturer is trying to save money by using less lube. So, if you buy one, check and lube if necessary.

TIP 3 – Do not buy an inexpensive (cheap) bike that has a rear shock. It costs the makers to provide this fancy, thus taking money from their bottom line. Therefore, they must make up for the loss anywhere they can. Which means the entire bike is furnished with the absolutely cheapest parts available.

TIP 4 – A light thin steel frame bike means less steel. Which means a bendable bike. Lighter is not necessarily better!

Bottom line: "You get what you pay for."

SPECIAL NOTE TO THE NEW CYCLIST: Remember that the more complex the bike, the more maintenance and know-how will be required of you, the owner. This is the case with buying a good bike that has both front and rear suspension.

ADDITIONAL NOTE: If you choose to buy a cheap bike, it is wise to check the wheels to make sure they are fully round and are not warped. Quality control can be iffy on cheap bikes. So, spin them and observe before you buy!

BUYING A USED BIKE

Sometimes there are unbelievable deals on used bikes in ads. But there are many things to consider first, before buying a used bike:

1) When you buy a used bike, you have no idea how its owner treated the bike—for example, whether that person used it as a jump bike or did a lot of curb hopping on it. Frame cracks are a concern, and so is metal fatigue. Always check for cracks, dents and ruffles on the frame, if your considering buying used. Chipped paint can be a telltale sign of frame cracking or damage. Frame damage cannot be fixed on the cheap and is specialized. So, never buy any bike that has a cracked, dented or ruffled frame, whether it's made of steel, aluminum, carbon or whatever. A damaged frame is dangerous. Pass it up!
2) You also have no idea the condition of its bearings. A bicycle has many sets of bearings that should be regularly cleaned and greased, or they will grind down and become uneven.
3) Worn parts will have to be replaced. Brake pads, tires, cables, chains, pedals, grips and again, bearings! These things cost money. And in the case of bearings, most

riders will probably want a bike mechanic to deal with them. Yes, more money!

4) Sometimes there will be a great deal on a nearly new bike, but the owner seems shady. He/she does not look much like a cyclist at all, and that should raise some suspicion. Why? Because people who don't ride bikes usually don't own them. This might be a case of bicycle theft. This is not too hard to spot—something just does not seem right. And its price might be too good to be true. It's a literal steal! Avoid this! Sometimes a stolen bike has passed hands many times. The seller and so-called owner bought it stolen from someone else, who bought it stolen also. Buying stolen stuff is a crime, so avoid this altogether. Buy it from a friend or someone you are sure of, if you need to buy used.

I am not a big fan of buying used. A bicycle is a personal thing and I like to know where it has been. And after considering all the above, I think you'll see buying new is always better, even if you must save some cash for a longer time.

TIP – Sometimes in a yard sale you will see some dusty bikes that were pulled out of a garage and put on sale just to clear some space. Here you can ask questions if you want to buy. The chances of buying a hot bike here is remote. Then there are thrift shops. Bikes here are used up discards. Yes, discards. Which means "to throw away."

NOTE: Buying a vintage bike can be extremely exciting! A vintage bike brings back the nostalgia of yesteryear. Most vintage bikes are just hanging around collecting dust in the garages of their owners, who just stopped biking. These can be a true treasure to those who appreciate the virtues, craftsmanship, and design of older bikes. I have a certain fascination with vintage mountain bikes. Bikes that were produced in the 80's and 90's have a lot of flair, color, and personality. And in many aspects, they were built better, which is why they are still around. These bikes are worth the extra cash to get them running and to reminisce.

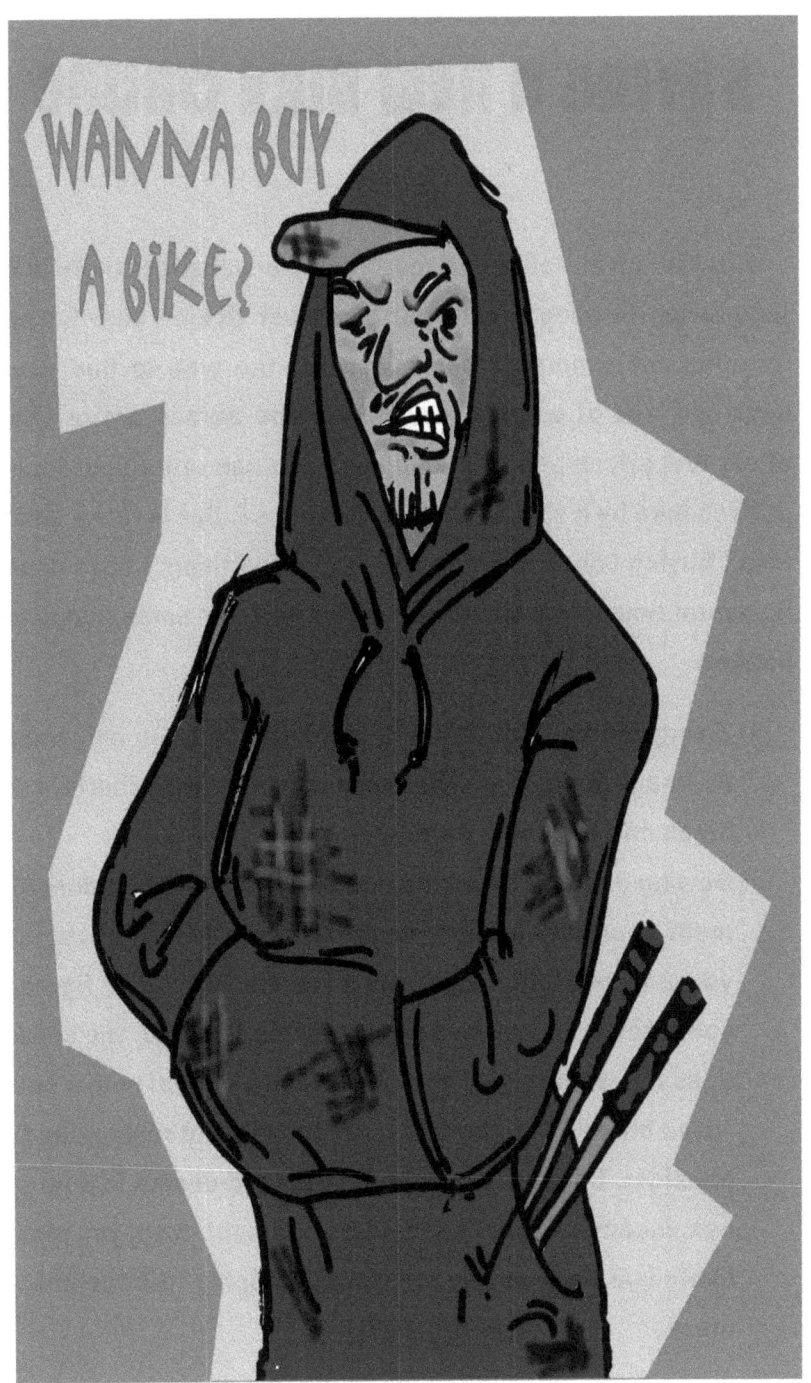

BUYING A NEW BIKE ONLINE

With the advent of online merchandise websites, there is a temptation to shop around for whatever tickles your fancy, bicycles not exempt. When searching the web to find your next new set of wheels, you may come across a site that offers low prices and free shipping! You can order your long-desired bike by a simple click of the mouse. But is this a good idea? Buying online is not in any way a bad thing. I have done it several times with satisfaction. But here are some things to ponder:

1) Sizing can be a bit difficult, given the fact you only have an image to look at. There are usually sizing charts, but bikes can run small or large.
2) Getting a refund on a bike you bought online, if it doesn't meet your satisfaction, might be an ordeal. Sometimes you are given the royal run-a-round. The seller figures you'll get tired and give up, and some do. Also, the seller does not want to give back the money, or deal with a now "used bike." Then there is repackaging and reshipping to consider. Being that a bike is large and comes in a large box, inconvenience is an understatement. Also, you most likely will have to pay for return shipping. It becomes a mess.

3) Shipping can damage a bike. If you buy online, your bike may be sent to you with scratches and dings. Sometimes heavy packages are placed on the bike's box, causing a rim to bend. These are common problems. And now you must deal with getting a refund or replacement.

4) Thrown off bike cable adjustments due to cable stretch is also an issue. But this should be expected, and doesn't require replacement, just simple adjustments. But there are other things that might have occurred in transit, like a bent rear derailleur hanger, that will permanently throw off the gear shifting. This is worthy of refund or replacement.

5) Getting in touch with the seller if there is a problem can be exceedingly difficult. They usually do not have a contact number to call on the website, and most likely you will never get to speak with a real person. So, you are forced to e-mail them. Good luck in getting a response.

All in all, buying online is fine if you know exactly what you are looking for and if you are proficient in performing your own adjustments. I have read many unfounded review complaints people have made about their online bike being a piece of junk, just because the shifters and brakes did not work properly when they received it. The real blame goes to the buyer for his/her lack of understanding and know-how. Of course, the shifters and brakes are not going to work perfectly, because the cables have stretched! They were fine-tuned when built and boxed, but after, the bike sat in a warehouse for months. This change in tuning is normal to a NEW bike, and is even a part of the break-in period after purchase, just like new strings on a guitar go out of tune. Making these adjustments is a part of owning and operating a bike, and you'll need to learn them!

As far as superficial damages like scratches are concerned, accepting them is probably a better option than going through the motions of replacement. A frame scratch sometimes makes a bike look rugged and seasoned. And on a mountain bike that's kinda cool! But not so on a frame ding. That weakens the frame and is not acceptable with a new purchase.

And as far as bent rims are concerned, it is best to get a refund or replacement if you do not know how to true them.

TIP – Before buying an online bike, carefully look at its specs and components. In fact, teach yourself how to understand specs and components. Carefully read the information and compare it to what is depicted. Magnify and study the image, too. Sometimes parts are changed out with similar or cheaper parts, thinking the buyer will not notice. Even the whole bike can be changed out to a cheaper bike. There are many things that a buyer can be cheated on if he/she does not look carefully.

ONE MAJOR SPEC YOU SHOULD NOTICE: Most bikes these days are sold with a lower toothed triple-ring crankset consisting of a 42/34/24 ratio or similar. Previous bikes were sold with a ratio of 48/38/28 or similar. The newer ratio is geared for hills, but falls truly short of any road riding. It simply does not allow you to ride with any speed, and you will wind out in frustration. This is a disappointing problem with today's bikes. It can only be remedied by changing out the crankset and ordering a new set having chainrings with the older ratio (Read more in Chapter 3, **CHAINRINGS**).

NOTE 1: While on the subject of cranksets, if the bike you're eyeballing for purchase has steel crankarms, then know that the cranks are cheap. If they are plastic-coated, then know they are plastic-coated steel. Doubly cheap!

NOTE 2: If you are going to buy a bike and do uphill riding, be sure to count the teeth of the biggest cog (on rear wheel). For uphill riding, it should have 34 teeth, or close to it. This number of teeth will allow you to climb very steep hills with relative ease.

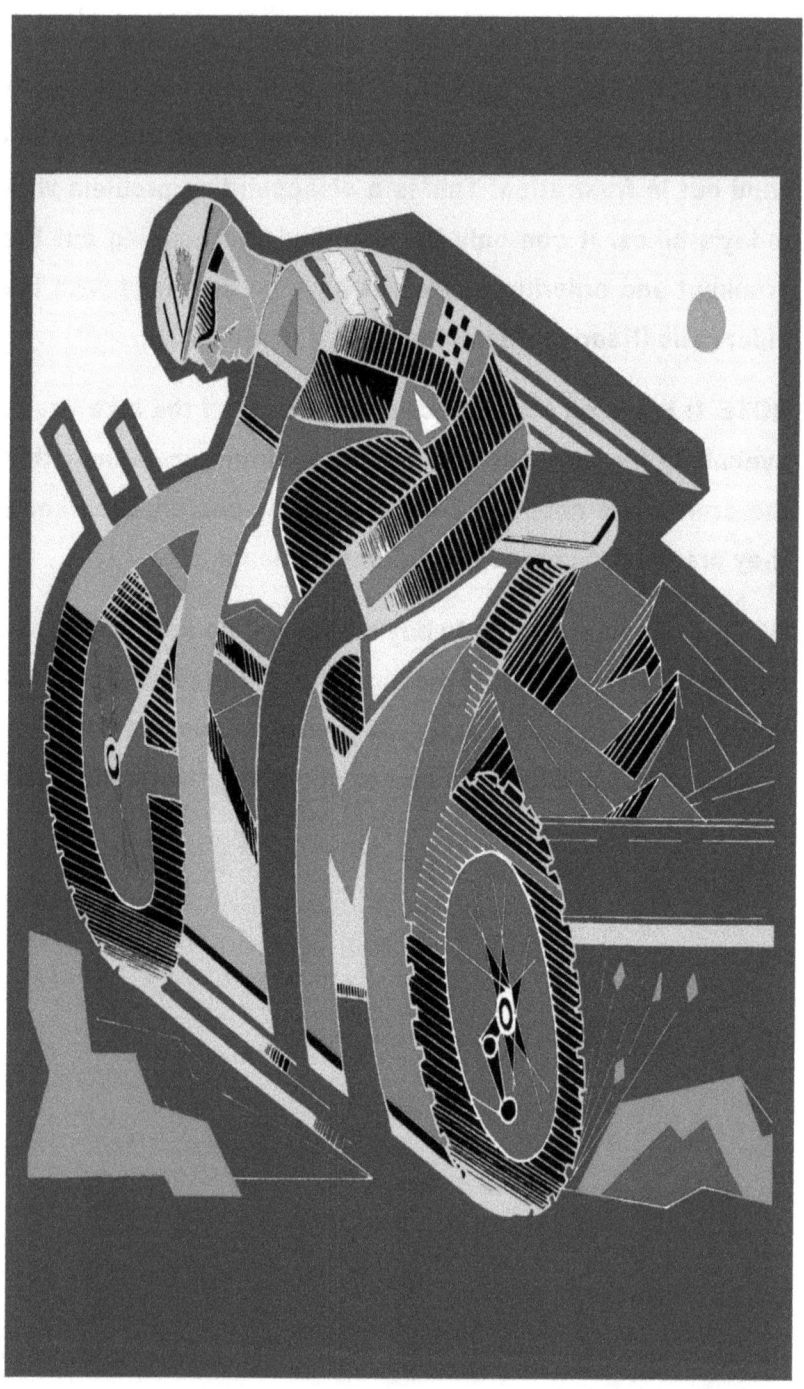

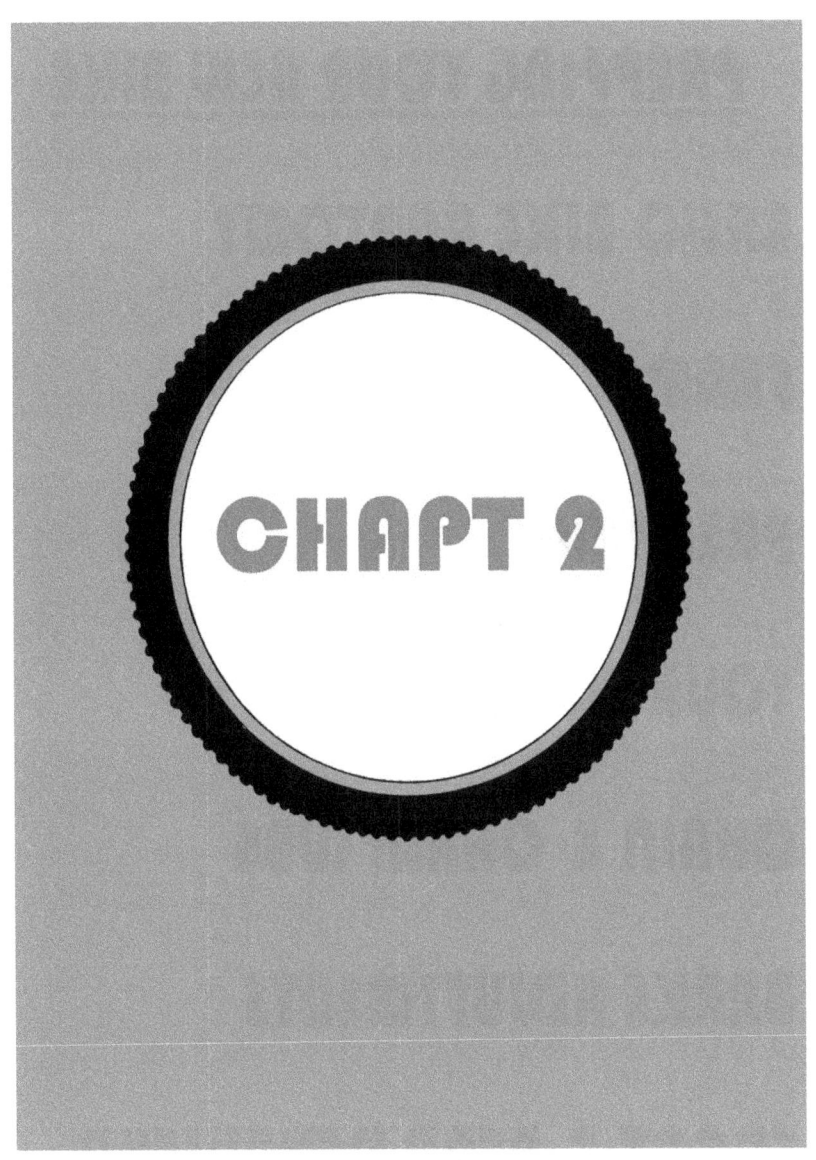

PREP SMART - THE ART OF PREPPING YOUR NEW BIKE

BASIC BIKE ANATOMY

FRAME

PREPPING

YOUR TOOLBOX

CHAIN & CHAIN LUBE

BRAKE ADJUSTMENTS

FRONT & REAR DERAILLEUR

QUICK TUNEUP

CHAINSTAY PROTECTOR

TIRE PRESSURE

BASIC BIKE ANATOMY

Here is a quick rundown of the anatomy of a bicycle. Knowing the names of the parts of a bike helps you communicate to the bike shop mechanic (if you have questions) **AND NOT SOUND STUPID!**

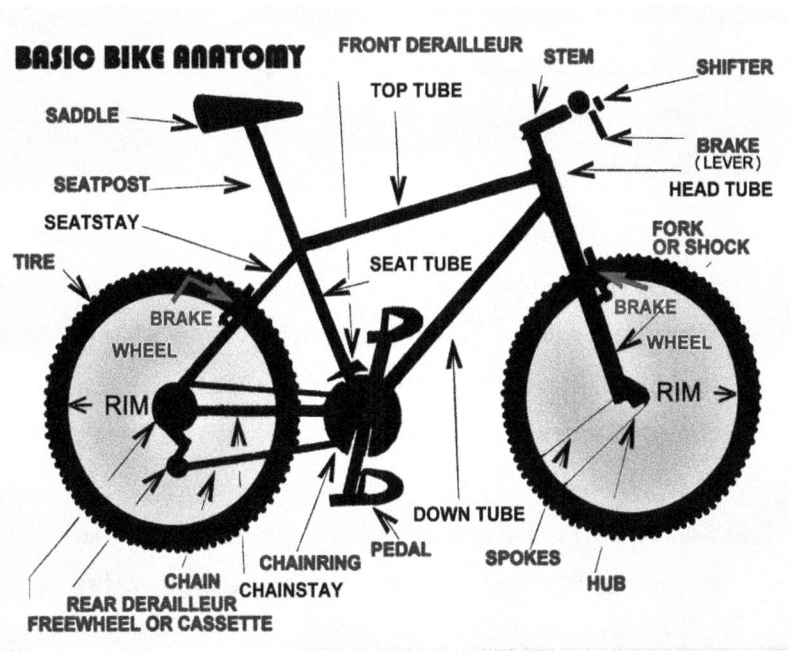

FRAME

The foremost part of a bike, which is the heart of a bike, is the frame. The quality, or lack thereof, of a frame can make or break a purchase. In choosing a bike, you must meticulously scrutinize this particular item. Reason being, all other parts can be swapped out, but the frame, is the bike. So, what are the things that must be taken into consideration?

1) Material: Aluminum or steel? An aluminum frame offers a lighter ride and will not rust if scratched. But you do feel vibrations more (not so much with bikes with fat tires and shocks). A steel frame on the other hand, dampens the road vibrations very well, but is heavier and rusts if scratched.

2) Bolt on options: Check the frame for cage braze-ons, also known as "bottle cage mounts," to attach water bottle cages. Also, check for mounts for a fork rack and a rear rack.

3) Welds: Inspect the welds to see if they are done well or have shoddy workmanship. Look for holes or gaps.

4) Detachable derailleur hanger: If a bike frame does not have a detachable rear derailleur hanger, it is a tell-tale sign of a not-so-good frame. A detachable derailleur hanger is a sacrificial part, designed to be replaced if

bent in the event your derailleur takes a big hit. This protects the frame. If the frame you buy does not carry one, a big hit to the derailleur will bend the permanent frame hanger and shifting will be affected and not fixable unless bent back. Bending it back may work on a steel frame, but not usually on an aluminum frame. Aluminum usually cracks if bent. You can identify a detachable derailleur hanger by looking at what the rear derailleur is mounted to. It should be mounted to a plate that is secured with a bolt to the frame, usually silver in color (but not always).

5) Color: Make sure before you buy a bike that you can live with the color. A lot of bikes come in neon colors, which are safer on the road by their visibility, but are an eye strain to look at. An extremely loud paint job is likely to make you hate looking at your bike over time.

SIZE MATTERS

Size is everything in a frame. The frame size needs to match your body's height. The usual way to get the right size is by using what is called "standover height." This is the distance from the ground to the very top of the top tube (at center). As you stand over the bike, there will be a space between your inseam and the top tube. This space determines the size of bike you need. Here are some rules for a good fit:

1) A road only bike should have about 2 inches of space.

2) An unpaved road/trail-only bike should have about 3 inches of space.

3) A mountain or off-road-only bike should have about 4 inches of space.

A bike that is a bit small can be made to fit a larger person by purchasing a longer stem and seatpost. But a large bike cannot be made to fit a smaller person. Different size bikes also have crank sizes that differ in length. Small crankarms (such as 170mm) on a bike can make pedaling feel cramped if you are tall (175mm crankarms are good for most). That's something to be aware of if you buy a bike with a small frame. So, be choosy, and get it right the first time.

TIP 1 – Don't let any bike salesman or any seller pressure you to buy a bike that is the wrong size for you, no matter how many goodies they offer with it, or how low they discount it. Sometimes a large bike has been sitting in a shop for a long time, and they just need to get rid of it. Large sizes are sometimes hard to sell. So, be aware of this, and don't be a sucker!

TIP 2 – You may be tempted to buy a bike that is not your size, because of a great sale, a yard sale find, or some other opportunity. These temptations come unexpectedly, and due to the urgency, make you buy compulsively. Don't give in to your whim, buy the bike that fits you. Use willpower!

NOTE: Frames usually come in the following sizes: xsmall, small, medium, large and xlarge.

THINGS YOU NEED TO KNOW APART FROM THE FRAME. WHAT IS A ...?

Bottom bracket - **the sealed cartridge or axle and bearings set that the cranks are attached to.**

Cassette - **the cluster of differing cogs the chain rides on that rotate on the back rear wheel hub. Cassettes do not contain a ratcheting drive in them.**

Freewheel - **the cluster of differing cogs that the chain rides on that rotate on the back rear wheel hub and contains its own ratcheting drive system and bearings.**

Cog or sprocket - **a single rounded, toothed gear that is separated by spacers held in a cluster (of many different size cogs) attached to the hub on the back wheel.**

Chainring - **a set of toothed rings a chain rides on that is connected to the cranks.**

Wheel quick-release - **a mechanism used to secure a wheel to the fork or dropouts. It consists of a quick-release skewer rod, two centering springs, and a cam lever on one side and an adjusting nut on the other.**

CASSETTE OR FREEWHEEL?

Most geared bikes are going to have either a cassette or a freewheel attached to the rear hub of the rear wheel. These two types of differing cog sets look almost identical. A cassette has no internal ratcheting mechanism. It depends on a ratcheting mechanism located in the wheel hub or freehub. A freewheel, on the other hand, has the ratcheting mechanism built into it. So, how do you tell if your bike has a cassette or a freewheel? Simply take your rear wheel off your bike. Remove the axle bolt (if bolt-on) or skewer rod (if quick-release). Locate the innermost splined tool fitting receptacle on the front. Now spin the cogs. If the splines move with the cogs, you have a cassette. If the splines do not move with the cogs, you have a freewheel. There may be exceptions to this rule, reason being, there are many different freewheel types. So, this identification test may not be fully reliable.

NOTE: Lower end bikes usually have a freewheel. Upper end bikes usually have a cassette.

YOU HAVE MADE AN EDUCATED DECISION AND HAVE PURCHASED YOUR NEW BIKE. WHAT NOW?

NOW IT'S TIME TO PREP YOUR RIDE.

HERE ARE SOME THINGS THAT NEED TO GET DONE AND CHECKED BEFORE YOU RIDE.

ALSO, SOME GOOD TIPS!

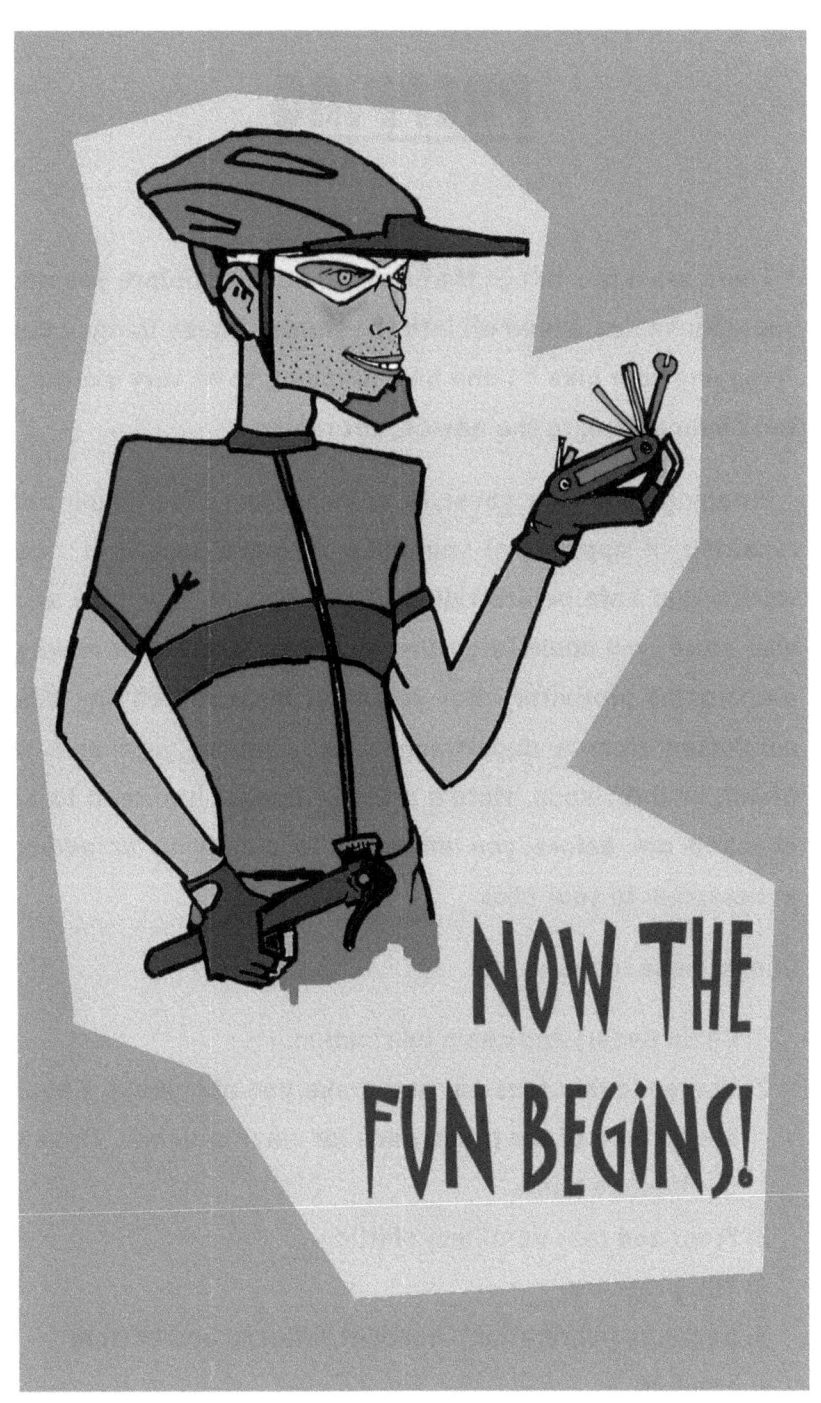

PREPPING

There are a few things that need to be done before you ride your mechanical steed off into the sunset. These things I call "prepping your bike." I find bike prepping to be very exciting. But chances are, to the novice, not really.

Prepping your bike consists of inspecting, fine-tuning and repairing (if applicable) your bike to make sure it is rideworthy and safe before riding. If you bought your bike at a bike store, you could forgo these checks (except for making a chainstay protector). But you must inspect well any bike purchased from a department store, online, yard sale, a friend, or thrift shop. Here's a list of things that need to be checked out before you move on to modifying or adding accessories to your bike.

Check these items:

1) Chain (wear) and chain lubrication.
2) Brakes (cable tension) and brake pad alignment. Check the surface of the brake pads for wear or debris. Grease the V-brake posts.
3) Front and rear derailleur shifting.
4) Tire pressure.
5) Bearings (lubrication): headset, wheels, and bottom bracket.

6) Spokes (loose spokes) and wheel straightness and roundness.

7) Crankarm bolts (needs to be tight).

NOTE 1: In addition to these things, check the tightness on all the bolts, including wheel quick-release levers. Also check the handlebar to front wheel alignment. (Other things like accessories are covered in Chapter 4).

NOTE 2: I consider prepping a bike as a time to get to know your bike. Whether the bike is new or used, it is still new to you, and needs to be explored. It's like a bike honeymoon, as a weird analogy. A person obviously gives a bike a quick look over before a purchase. But after, in prepping it, you get to really know your bike more thoroughly.

Some benefits of prepping are:

- It makes you aware of any manufacturing flaws in your bike (if new), allowing you to return it early, while you can.
- You will also know the specific tools to carry along with you on your ride, having identified your bike's repair requirements.
- It will help you to identify specific types of extra parts to store in your toolbox for future repairs.
- In the case of a used bike, it helps to identify poorly done repairs and wrong parts added.
- Most importantly, it makes your bike safe to ride.

As a whole, prepping helps you take ownership of your bike because familiarity makes it more personal to you. And a bike is a personal thing!

NOTE 3: Your bike will need a chainstay protector. More on this later in this chapter under **CHAINSTAY PROTECTOR**.

YOUR TOOLBOX

A cyclist should have a special toolbox just for his/her bike. This toolbox is separate from any household toolbox in that it has only tools needed to repair a bike. These tools are not the tools that you carry with you on a ride, but a larger and more extensive set that you keep at home. I will give a list of the most basic bike repair tools needed for most repairs and adjustments. I will also give a list of things other than tools that are needed and should be in your box. Having a bike toolbox will make you more organized in repairing your bike, keeping you from having to search the garage for the tools and items you need. It also makes you feel more confident in your repairs by having the right tools for the job. (In addition to this toolbox, you will need a bike stand).

THE MOST BASIC TOOLS FOR THE AVERAGE CYCLIST (BASED ON A NEWER TYPE BIKE):

1) Chain tool (chain breaker) with chain hook.
2) Cable and housing cutter with crimping tool.
3) Allen wrenches (make sure there is a size for the crank bolt).
4) Spoke wrench (size for your wheel).
5) Crankarm extractor.
6) Pipe cutter (for trimming down handlebars).
7) Basic pliers.

8) Large pump with a gauge.
9) Cartridge retainer ring tool.
10) Adjusting crescent wrench.
11) Rubber mallet.
12) Flathead and Phillips screwdrivers.
13) Scissors.
14) Pedal wrench.
15) Freewheel remover.
16) Tire levers.
17) File.
18) Chain whip.
19) Chain wear indicator gauge tool.
20) Chain master link pliers.

OTHER THINGS NEEDED IN YOUR TOOLBOX:

- **Black electrical tape (this may contain lead and other toxins). Wash hands after handling.**
- **Black zip-ties of differing sizes.**
- **Velcro (black) self-adhesive roll.**
- **Pieces of tire tube.**
- **Rubber gloves and mask.**
- **Extra aluminum cable end caps (these occasionally fall off).**
- **Extra end plugs for handlebars (these too occasionally fall off).**
- **Patches (2 types).**
- **Snap-on-cleaner for chain cleaning.**
- **Extra tube valve caps.**

- Paper towels.

NOTE 1: A cyclist should have five different types of bicycle lubrication in his/her repair kit/toolbox:

- A general all-purpose oil (for creaking parts).
- A chain lube (for chains only).
- Bicycle grease (for bearings).
- WD-40 (for stuck parts).

NOTE 2: There are four things that are indispensable to the cyclist and should be mentioned twice. These items are for all your tinkering and modification needs, especially mounting items to your handlebars. They are:

- Self-adhesive Velcro strips (black).
- Black tape (may contain lead). Use it where you're not going to touch it, and wash your hands after handling.
- Zip-ties.
- Tire tube slivers (pieces).

CHAIN & CHAIN LUBE

Many bikes out of the store have a protective coating of some sort on the chain. This is the case if you notice the chain feels kind of sticky and less bendable than it should. It is advisable to clean and apply the appropriate chain lube to the chain after purchase or following a few rides.

Major department stores carry a decent line of bike products, including chain lube, and some do sell some of the main brands that bike stores carry. The store will have several types of chain lube that you can match to the conditions you will be riding your bike through. They may also sell a plastic snap-on cleaner gadget that has wheel brushes and a reservoir for liquid cleaner to clean your chain. It usually comes with its own liquid cleaner. When the liquid cleaner runs out, you can use a bottle of "Simple Green" as a replacement. It is good to use a mat or newspapers under your bike when you clean your chain, as it can get messy. Chain cleaning and lubing are routine functions of owning a bike. Do both once a month and as your riding dictates.

HOW TO CLEAN

To clean your chain, you can either use the spray and wipe method (with Simple Green or a similar product) or the snap-on cleaner method. Put on some rubber gloves before you begin doing either, and like I said, use a mat or some newspapers under your bike.

SPRAY AND WIPE METHOD

Put gloves on, then spray the chain (avoid spraying cleaner on frame and tires) and let soak for a few minutes. Then wipe clean with paper towels till the towels no longer have any black residue on them. After cleaning, let the chain sit for a while till the inner pins and rollers are fully dry. Then apply the chain lube (start at master link) generously (avoid dripping lube on frame, brake pads and tires) and let it sit all night. In the morning, get paper towels and wipe off the chain. Chain lube can attract dirt, so make sure you wipe off any excess lube. The lube should be in the inside, not outside, of the chain.

SNAP-ON CLEANER METHOD

This method depends on the version of snap-on cleaner that you buy, so its instructions may vary from device to device. But generally, the device's lid is opened, and the reservoir is filled with liquid cleaner to the fill line. Then the chain is sandwiched between the lid and bottom portion between its wheels and locked closed by a wire latch. There is another part that attaches to the rear derailleur to keep it in position.

Then the cranks are spun till the chain is clean. The lid is opened, and the chain is wiped clean and left to dry. After, chain lube is applied (avoid dripping lube on frame, brake pads and tires) and left to sit overnight. In the morning, the excess chain lube is wiped with paper towels. Use gloves here too.

I find the best way to apply chain lube is to place a drop of lube on each chain roller. Start lubing at the master link to identify where you began, so that you will know where to stop. This practice conserves chain lube and is tidy.

TIP 1 – Do not use motor oil, baby oil, or WD-40 as chain lubricants. Use only a chain lube designed for bicycles and their conditions. However, you can use WD-40 to loosen stiff links (lube after).

TIP 2 – If you purchase a new chain, understand that it too will have a protective coating on it. This sticky factory lube will need to be cleaned off and the chain will need to be lubed with the appropriate lube. Read the instructions that are on the package.

TIP 3 – Mechanical advice about chains: While riding, the combinations of gearing you choose should be thought out to keep your chain in as straight a line as possible. In other words, don't ride with your chain in a straining and bending position, such as with the chain on the large chainring and the largest cog or with the smallest chainring and the smallest cog. These are extreme positions. This is not good for the drivetrain altogether. Choose a straight and smooth path for your chain.

TIP 4 – Carry a small length of chain with your tools as you ride (more on what items to bring along with you in Chapter 5, **HYDRATION PACK-TOOLS**).

TIP 5 – Over time the pins and rollers on a chain become worn, and thus the spacing between rollers increases. This increase of spacing in the chain causes wear on the parts the chain rides on, like the chainrings and cogs. So a chain should be replaced about every 1,000 miles. This will prevent premature wear on your chainrings and cogs.

TIP 6 – Stiff chain links can be freed by gently flexing the stiff point laterally back and forth.

TIP 7 – If you don't have a chain wear indicator tool, you can still tell if your chain needs to be replaced by simply holding a 12-inch ruler to it. Hold the starting 1-inch mark to a chain pin center. The end of the 12-inch mark should stop at the center of another pin. If it is off by as much as 1/8-inch, it needs to be replaced.

NOTE: While on the subject of the chain and chain cleaning, keep in mind that your bike's whole drivetrain needs to be cleaned regularly. What is a drivetrain, you might ask? Your bike's drivetrain consists of a freewheel or cassette (cogs), chainrings, chain, derailleurs and pedals. And these get dirty often. So, clean these along with the chain. Your drivetrain's longevity depends on the upkeep of your chain.

BRAKE ADJUSTMENTS

If you buy your new bike from a department store or online, it's almost a given that your brakes are not going to be working sharply right upon purchase. Do not worry, there is nothing wrong with the bike! The brakes have been adjusted correctly from the manufacturer, but there is the usual cable stretch (mentioned earlier) and bad bike rebuilding that might have thrown off their adjustment. They just need some simple readjusting.

Being that brake adjusting is somewhat a recurrent task, every bike rider should be very familiar with his/her brakes. Unless you like running to the bike store for everything and wasting money. This book is not so much a "how to book," but a book to bring to awareness what riders need to know most. There are many instructional videos online that will fortify your knowledge on the topic of brakes.

That being said, brake adjusting on a bike is not rocket science. But no doubt, something every rider will have to learn, regardless of his/her skill level. Why? Simply because, like I said, it is somewhat a recurrent task (especially on cheap bikes), and often enough, must be addressed on the road. That means, by yourself! And clearly, braking is vital to riding safety. So, a good understanding is necessary.

When you first buy a bike in a bike store, you are good-to-go, as far as any brake adjustments are concerned, and all other adjustments for that matter. Because all bike store bikes must be in proper working order before the bike goes out the door. But, in about a month, there will be additional adjustments needed (to both brakes and derailleurs), as cable stretch happens to all new bikes regardless of where they are purchased. Fortunately, in time, cable stretch will decrease, and cable adjustments will be less frequent. Having that to look forward to, the downside is there is more to brakes than just cable tension, as I will now get into. Now let's get into the basics of V-brakes and some tips.

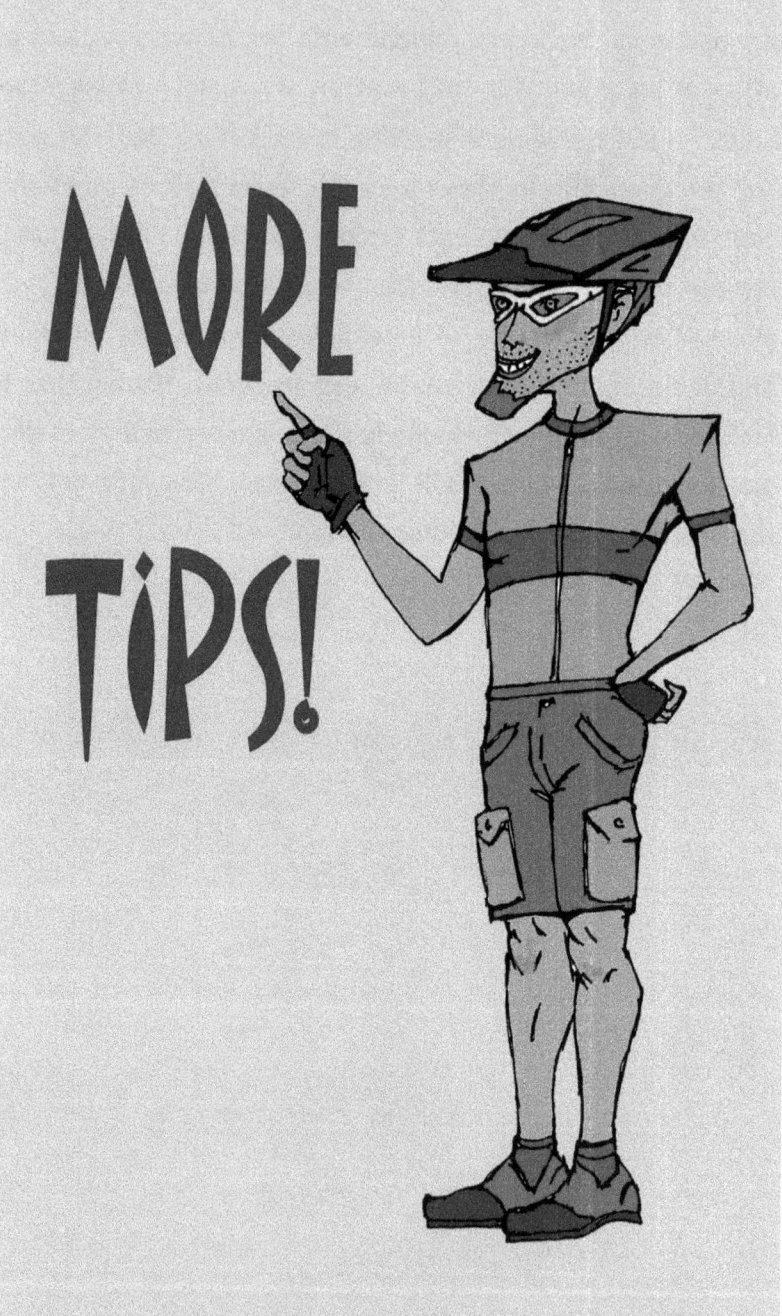

V-BRAKES

V-brakes are powerful and reliable bicycle braking mechanisms. They consist of two brake arms, pads, cable noodle, noodle holder, anchor bolt and tension screws.

Adjusting V-brakes involves proper cable tension from the brake lever to V-brake, orientation of brake arms, brake pad alignment, and smooth and lubed cable path. Here's the breakdown:

1) Brake cable tension should be as such as to not allow the brake lever to touch the grip. But breaking should begin at about half-way.
2) The brake arm's orientation should be upwardly straight, and the spacing between the rim and brake pad on each side should be equal. Straightness and spacing are done by adjusting the tension screws located on the side of each arm. These two tension screws (one on each side) serve to add or subtract spring tension, causing each arm to lean in one direction or another. By adding or subtracting tension to one side, both brake arms will move together (since they are connected via cable) in either direction, thus achieving proper spacing. You may have to add tension to one side and loosen tension on the other, to find the correct spacing, proper tension, and straightness. It is a balancing act.
3) Brake pads should be situated on the rim where the whole pad contacts the rim in a flat manner. No part of

the pad should be above the upper edge of the rim where it would contact the tire and wear into it. Nor should the pad extend beyond the lower edge of the rim where it would lessen braking power and deform the pad. Pads should be flat on the rim. But, due to chronic braking squeal, sometimes the pads orientation needs to be changed from parallel to SLIGHTLY pointing to the rim. This is called "toeing in" and is done to both brake pads. This eliminates the squealing sound brake pads can make and does not affect braking. Remember, the brake pads should angle to the front of the bike.

4) Brake cables should be free of rust, lubed and have an unobstructed path.

TIP 1 – Check your brake pads regularly. Look for embedded metal shavings or rocks. If found, pick them out and clean the pad. If you hear a scraping sound while you brake, stop immediately and inspect your brake pads. A scraping sound means there is something stuck on the pad. This will scratch into your rim. A small pocketknife may be needed to remove any stuck debris. So, carry one.

TIP 2 – Sometimes one side of a brake pad will rub against the rim of your wheel, making a thumping sound as you ride. This means your wheel is not fully centered. This can happen after fixing a flat, or any time you remove your wheel and put it back on. If a brake pad is rubbing and the wheel needs centering: Simply loosen the wheel quick-release locking lever and adjust the wheel to center. Then, retighten the wheel quick-release locking lever. Rotate your wheel to make sure it's centered and not getting rubbed. A warped rim can also cause a brake pad to rub.

TIP 3 – When adjusting the V-brakes, and you need the pads to be held flat against the rim, do this: Simply take a rubber band and pull it over the corresponding grip and brake lever and let it go. This will keep the lever in a braking clench, and pads flat on the rim, allowing you to adjust the pads and tighten the bolts with relative ease. You can also release the tension springs from the brake arms for more ease.

TIP 4 – For crisp responsive braking, regularly clean and grease the posts that the brake arms swing on and are bolted to. These often become dirty and dry, needing cleaning and fresh grease. Remember, grease only the posts, not the bolts or inner threads.

TIP 5 – Upon removal of each brake arm (for post cleaning and greasing), you will unseat the brake's tension spring on both sides. Each tension spring has one curved tip of it inserted in one of three holes located at the base of the post. If you don't remember which of the three holes the spring tip was inserted into, it is usually the middle one.

Tip 6 – "Toeing in" the brake pads is usually a last resort to stopping chronic brake squeal. Remember that brake pads and rims become glazed over at times, and for simple reasons as getting them wet, pads especially. Cleaning the rim and dulling the pad is the usual remedy. So, wipe pads and rims clean with alcohol first and check braking. If that does not work, lightly scuff the surface of the pad with a file to dull the surface. This usually does the trick. If not, then you can proceed to "toeing in" the pads. And if these don't work, you can also lightly resurface the rim braking surface with an emery cloth.

NOTE 1: When scuffing the pads, use a file and not sandpaper. Sandpaper granules can break off and imbed into the pad surface. The granules will no doubt scratch into the rim. Also, use a file that is lightly coarse, so as not to remove too much of the pad surface. You only want to dull the surface.

NOTE 2: Wipe your rims and pads from time to time with alcohol to clean off any residual brake pad material and glazing.

FRONT & REAR DERAILLEUR

On any given ride as I pass other cyclists, I will hear that all-too-familiar sound of a chain grinding against a derailleur cage, or the maddening chatter of a chain stuck in mid-shift. Are these riders oblivious? Or are they just ignoring these truly irritating noises, hoping they will magically go away? My guess is that they just don't want to deal with their bike's derailleurs, or they have tried and failed! Why? Because derailleurs are complicated!

Every cyclist and bike owner who has a bike with gears will have to deal with adjusting their derailleurs sooner or later. The choices being, they can delegate it to the shop, fix it themselves, or just tolerate the sounds of their bike begging for help as their derailleur cage gets worn away. Or they can hope the benevolent bike fairy will come flying through their window at night and perform a bike tune-up for them.

Since derailleurs are intimidating and adjusting them multi-faceted, I will endeavor to demystify them, and break down adjusting them to simple steps.

BASIC 101

On a bike, the front and rear derailleur will often fall out of adjustment due to cable stretch or anything that causes the cable tension to change. Today's shifting systems are quite sensitive, and a tiny amount of cable slackening can go a long way in causing chain chatter and rough shifting. Tuning is accomplished by the cable barrels situated on the shifter for the front derailleur and on the rear derailleur for the back.

And beyond cable tension, there are derailleur limit screws. And a person, no doubt, will have to deal with these screws in addition to cables for adjustments. Because slack cables are not the only thing that causes malfunctioning shifts. It is these two complexities together that make derailleurs the scary little mechanisms that they are.

LIMIT SCREWS

Derailleurs have two limit screws on them. These are marked with an "H" for high-gear and an "L" for low-gear. They limit how far in or out a derailleur can move. They also set the baseline for shifting. Adjusting these limit screws keeps the chain from falling off both sides of the cog or chainrings (over-shifting).

TIP 1 – Just remember, as you look from the rear of your bike forward, that "L" means "left", and corresponds to adjustments on both derailleurs to the left side of the gears.

TIP 2 – When it comes to setting limit screws, remember that the front derailleur needs the "L" screw setting done first, and after that the "H". And on the rear derailleur, it is the opposite. The "H" screw is set first, then the "L" screw is set after. Setting limit screws in order is important, as derailleur adjusting is done in steps.

QUICK TUNE-UP

FRONT DERAILLEUR

FIRST, HERE ARE THE BASICS AND RULES:

1) All adjustments are done with cable tensioning. The limit screws only stop the derailleurs at a point.
2) The left shifter only controls the shift to the middle chainring (triple-ring crankset).
3) The shifters are the brain, not the derailleurs.

NOW YOU NEED TO DO A PRE-ADJUSTMENT INSPECTION. CHECK THESE ITEMS FIRST BEFORE DOING ANYTHING:

1) The front derailleur's cage should rest at 1/16-inch or 2mm above the largest chainring's teeth.
2) The front derailleur's cage should be parallel to the chainrings.
3) The front derailleur's cable should be clean, lubed, and move easily.
4) Look for any bent chainrings and straighten, if needed (gently hit with a rubber mallet or bend into position with an adjustable wrench).
5) Make sure the chain is good.
6) Make sure your rear derailleur is tuned (firstly before adjusting the front derailleur) and is not bent.

SCREW SETTING (TRIPLE-RING CRANKSET)

STEP 1: DETACH CABLE

1) Put bike on a stand.
2) Shift chain to smallest chainring and biggest cog.
3) Completely detach the front derailleur cable.
4) Turn shifter barrel all the way in, then out two turns.

STEP 2: INNER CAGE SPACING ("L" SCREW SETTING)

1) Spin cranks and adjust the spacing between the chain and the left side of the inner cage. Turn "L" limit screw just enough to where the scraping stops (1/32-inch or 1mm) or as small as possible.
2) Reattach the derailleur cable, tension the cable to where it is slightly taut.
3) Test to see if there is over-shift (inward chain dropping). Shift up and down from the smallest chainring to the middle.
4) "L" screw is set.

STEP 3: OUTER CAGE SPACING ("H" SCREW SETTING)

1) Shift chain to largest chainring and smallest cog.
2) Run a quick shifting check. Add or subtract tension as needed. Then go back to large chainring and small cog.

3) Spin cranks and adjust the spacing between the chain and right side of the inner cage. Turn "H" limit screw just enough to where the scraping stops (1/32-inch or 1mm) or as small as possible. You can assist the movement of the derailleur with your thumb (while you turn the screw), if it is too tight (to avoid stripping the screw).
4) While spinning cranks, test to see if there is over-shift (outward chain dropping). Shift fast and hard to the middle chainring and back to the largest. Stop spinning cranks and push hard on the shifter lever as far as it goes. Check for outward derailleur cage movement. There should not be any.
5) Further fine-tuning is now done with cable tensioning.
6) "H" screw is set.

STEP 4: TESTING SCREW ADJUSTMENTS AND ADJUSTING CABLE TENSION (FINE-TUNING)

1) Shift chain to a middle cog, as this is the ideal cog to check the adjustments.
2) Shift chain (from the chainrings) from large to the middle, middle to the small. Then in reverse, up and down. If there is any hesitation, adjust with cable tension. Add or subtract cable tension as needed.
3) Go through as many rear cog and chainring combinations as you can. Avoid large chainring and large cog, small chainring and small cog combinations, both in checking the adjustments and in riding in general (mentioned

earlier). The drivetrain was not designed to handle these combinations. Subsequently, any tuning done in these combinations will not work and will mess things up. There will be chain rub in these combinations due to the extreme chain positioning.

4) Go for a test ride.

5) The tricky part: When the limit screws are set correctly, any adjustments thereafter are done with cable tension. And ideally, after getting the right tension, your adjustments should be done. But, because there is strong force applied to the cranks while pedaling, there may be lateral flex to the crankset. And as a result, chain rub may happen in the large chainring, making some compensation necessary to the original setting. So, in addition to cable tensioning, the use of further slight "H" screw tuning and other means MAY have to be employed to counteract this lateral flex to get the shifting right. And, by the way, make any "H" limit screw tuning at this point, in small ¼ turns.

HERE ARE THOSE OTHER MEANS TO GETTING THE RIGHT SHIFTING:

1) You can "toe-in" or "toe-out" the derailleur cage. That means slightly turning the derailleur cage inward or outward. Yes, this is a contradiction to **PRE-ADJUSTMENT INSPECTION** rule 2, but it is needed at times. But start with a parallel positioning first.

2) Another trick you can do is adding a small washer to the back of the cage to the screw where it joins the cage ends.

3) And another is to slightly bend the derailleur's nose in or out.

NOTE: I find front derailleur adjusting to be a balancing act of screw setting, cable tensioning, and adding some other tricks to get it right. To me, it starts off as science and ends up as an art. But in the end, experience wins the day. Set the screws, adjust the tension, and see what you're left with. The key to overall front derailleur adjusting is getting that tight spacing between the inner cage and chain on both sides. If the whole process overwhelms you, you can always go to the shop to get it done or wait for the benevolent bike fairy. It's not expensive. The rear derailleur, on the other hand, to me is more straight forward.

REAR DERAILLEUR ADJUSTMENT: QUICK METHOD

Assuming the limit screws are properly set, and the bike is somewhat new or undamaged, here is the quickest and easiest way to dial in the rear derailleur adjustment:

1) Put the bike on a stand. Shift the chain to the smallest cog of the rear wheel and in the front to the largest chainring.

2) Loosen ALL tension out of the rear derailleur cable, making it slack (twist tension barrel located on derailleur to accomplish this).
3) Shift the right shifter lever one click, which would be for the second to the smallest cog. Since there is no tension or motion, the chain will not shift. You'll still be on the smallest cog.
4) Start spinning the crankarms and at the same time start tightening the tension by twisting the barrel. When the chain shifts to the second cog up from the bottom, turn the barrel about 1-3 more half turns (experiment what works for your bike). This should complete the rear adjustment.

SETTING REAR DERAILLEUR "H" (HIGH) AND "L" (LOW) SCREWS

On the rear derailleur, each limit screw is set by aligning vertically the derailleur guide pulley (top derailleur pulley) to the large or small cog (depending on which screw is being set). This is the big picture.

STEP 1: "H" SCREW SETTING (BASELINE)

1) Put bike on a bike stand.
2) Shift chain to small cog/large chainring.

3) Detach the derailleur cable altogether. Any cable tension will interfere with getting the right screw setting.
4) Align the derailleur guide pulley straight with the smallest cog. If your derailleur is old and the spring is worn, you can go 1mm past the outside of the small cog to compensate for the weak spring. Turn the "H" screw till guide pulley lines up with cog center. Further refine the tuning by spinning the cranks while gingerly turning "H" screw left and right till all chain chatter stops. There should be no chatter from the chain when fully centered. Turning the screw clockwise or counterclockwise will cause the derailleur to move left or right (in or out).
5) "H" screw is set.

STEP 2: "L" SCREW SETTING

1) Shift chain to the smallest chainring. Now with your hand (while spinning cranks) push the derailleur (chain will follow) to the largest cog.
2) Stop spinning cranks. Continue to hold the derailleur secure in position, pushing on it outward left as far as it goes. Align the guide pulley to the large cog by turning "L" screw (while spinning cranks again) till centered and without chatter. You can have someone assist and spin the cranks while you finish adjusting the screw. You will feel and see the derailleur slowly move inward and outward as you turn the screw. Again, turning screw clockwise or counterclockwise will cause the derailleur to move left or right (in or out).

3) Let go of the derailleur and spin cranks. The derailleur will return the chain back to the small cog. Shift chain to large chainring. Turn derailleur cable barrel all the way in, then 2 turns out. Reattach cable and tighten back cable till taut.
4) Lastly, press hard on the right shifter thumb lever and observe if there is any movement (play) by the derailleur. There should not be any. Spin cranks and check for chain chatter and over-shift.
5) "L" screw is set.

STEP 3: ADJUST CABLE TENSION (FINE-TUNING)

1) You can use the rear derailleur quick tune-up method now, or go to the next step.
2) Shift to middle chainring. Now shift one cog up and down at a time (while spinning cranks) and test shifting. Add or subtract cable tension upon hearing any chain chatter on each shift. Find the happy medium. Tune all the way up to the second to last cog. Use ¼ turns.
3) Press hard on the right thumb shifter again to see if there is any movement by the derailleur (as newly added cable tension might have changed the fine-tuning). Spin cranks and check for chain drop (over-shift).
4) Test ride the bike.

TIP 1 – If for any reason the rear derailleur will not adjust correctly, you may have a bent rear derailleur hanger. Even the slightest bend in the hanger can cause shifting problems.

The bend may be barely visible, too. This problem is identified when the shifting problems occur in the cogs that are in the center of the freewheel/cassette. A bent rear derailleur hanger will need to be straightened or replaced in order to complete any adjusting. If the derailleur hanger is of a flat plate type (as some can have a fancy design), remove it, and lay it flat on a table. Any warping will be easily visible. A warped hanger can be bent back to shape with a special tool.

TIP 2 – Clean and oil your rear derailleur pulleys (jockey wheels) on a regular basis. Caked-on road dirt will accumulate on the sides of them, and they will make an irritating chirping sound if they are dry.

TIP 3 – Cogs need to be cleaned at times. They will collect crud, too. You can use an old dish scrubbing brush to do this.

TIP 4 – In adjusting any derailleur, DO NOT go in all willy-nilly, turning screws and shifter barrels, thinking you'll get it right somehow. You will create an adjusting mess and a truly frustrating situation. Especially if you do not know what you are doing. Work cautiously and methodically, not haphazardly!

NOTE 1: On setting the "H" and "L" screws (rear derailleur), always strive to lean the adjustments biased towards the cogs. This will make it less likely the chain will drop in either direction.

NOTE 2: The rear derailleur has a tensioning screw at the rear of it. This is the B-tension adjustment. This screw is used to add or subtract space between the large cog and guide pulley.

Go to the largest cog and small chainring (granny gear). Spin cranks to check if the cog is hitting the rear derailleur pulley. This can happen if the chain is too small or if the screw is not adjusted right. If it makes contact, adjust screw to add more space between the cog and pulley. There should be 11-13mm space between, or as specified by the manufacturer.

NOTE 3: Any chain chatter while shifted on the large or small cog is most likely a rear derailleur limit screw maladjustment. This can be fixed by following the "L" or "H" screw setting instructions.

NOTE 4: Derailleur adjusting can vary from mechanic to mechanic. There will be slight variations in techniques and as to what comes first, even though the basic idea is the same. This can be confusing, especially if you are trying to learn from them. But the overall big picture of understanding both front and rear derailleur adjusting is pretty simple. Set the limit screws, and the rest is fine-tuning the cable tension. Demystified!

CHAINSTAY PROTECTOR

One thing I always do when I get a new bike is to make a chainstay protector. The chainstay is the part of the frame that receives the most abuse by a whipping chain, even with normal riding. Nothing makes a bike look shabby more quickly than a scratched up and pitted chainstay. So, to make one, find an old tube that has had its day. Cut off a segment of it, roughly the size of the chainstay. Then, cut it long ways and wash out the powder inside it. Then, place it long ways around the stay and overlap the excess. With black electrical tape, fasten it in position. Lastly, take black zip-ties and secure tightly. You can remove the black tape (if you choose) once the zip-ties are in position. This will render the whipping chain powerless to cause damage, and will make your ride less noisy. You can also wrap the chainstay with a cut inner tube in the same way you wrap handlebar tape.

TIP – Even though some bikes already come with a thin protective sticker on the chainstay, it is still necessary and prudent to make your own and place it over the existing one.

NOTE: Steel frames will rust where the paint has been chipped off, more reason to protect this part of the frame.

TIRE PRESSURE

Tire service is a routine task every bike rider should be proficient in. In fact, every time you take your bike out, you should check your tires first. It is a given that your new bike, when bought, might not have the proper tire pressure, or what is properly known as PSI (pounds per square inch). There are recommended pressures that are prescribed on the tire wall for every tire. Tire pressure is one of those things that is a personal preference, and something you tweak depending on road conditions and your preference. However, do not go above the recommended maximum pressure stated, or KABOOM!

As for me, I normally run a riding pressure that is generally below the stated tire pressure. On my hybrid bike, for example, I have a certain PSI that I use for what I call a soft ride and one for a hard ride. Both are well below the stated pressure and work well. Depending on the roads I choose to ride, I decide which one will suit for the day. The city streets in my city are loaded with uneven patchy areas, whereas the recommended standard high pressure stated on my tires, when followed, make for a jolty and brutal ride. So, I had to adjust. It has taken some trial and error to find these sweet spot pressures. The takeaway is that tire pressures are somewhat dictated by the roads which you ride.

As for recording these numbers, I have written them down on my large pump, so I don't forget and can meter out the exact PSI every time. I also have the PSI I use most dialed in on my pump gauge indicated by the red dial needle that is for that purpose. So, it is necessary to buy a pump that has a pressure gauge (and one with a red dial needle). I have learned that an exact standard is vastly better than just feeling the tire, the "squeeze test." This is especially true on a high-pressure hybrid. But it does go for mountain bikes as well. You should own a large pump with a gauge and a small mini pump attached to every bike you own.

TIP – Low tire PSI can cause what is known as a "snake bite flat." It appears as two holes on the tube as if it has been bitten by a snake. This happens when you have low tire pressure and hit something hard, directly. Your tire will compress to such a degree that the sides of the rim will dig into the tube and cause a blow-out. A double flat! Prolonged low tire pressure while riding can also damage a rim and shred or crack the sides of a tire. So, keep your tires well within reasonable pressures.

NOTE: Do not inflate tires or store in an enclosed area a bike that has its tires fully pressurized. Tires can blow and cause air pressure to abruptly increase, and may cause damage to the ears. Inflate tires outside and lower tire pressure before storing indoors.

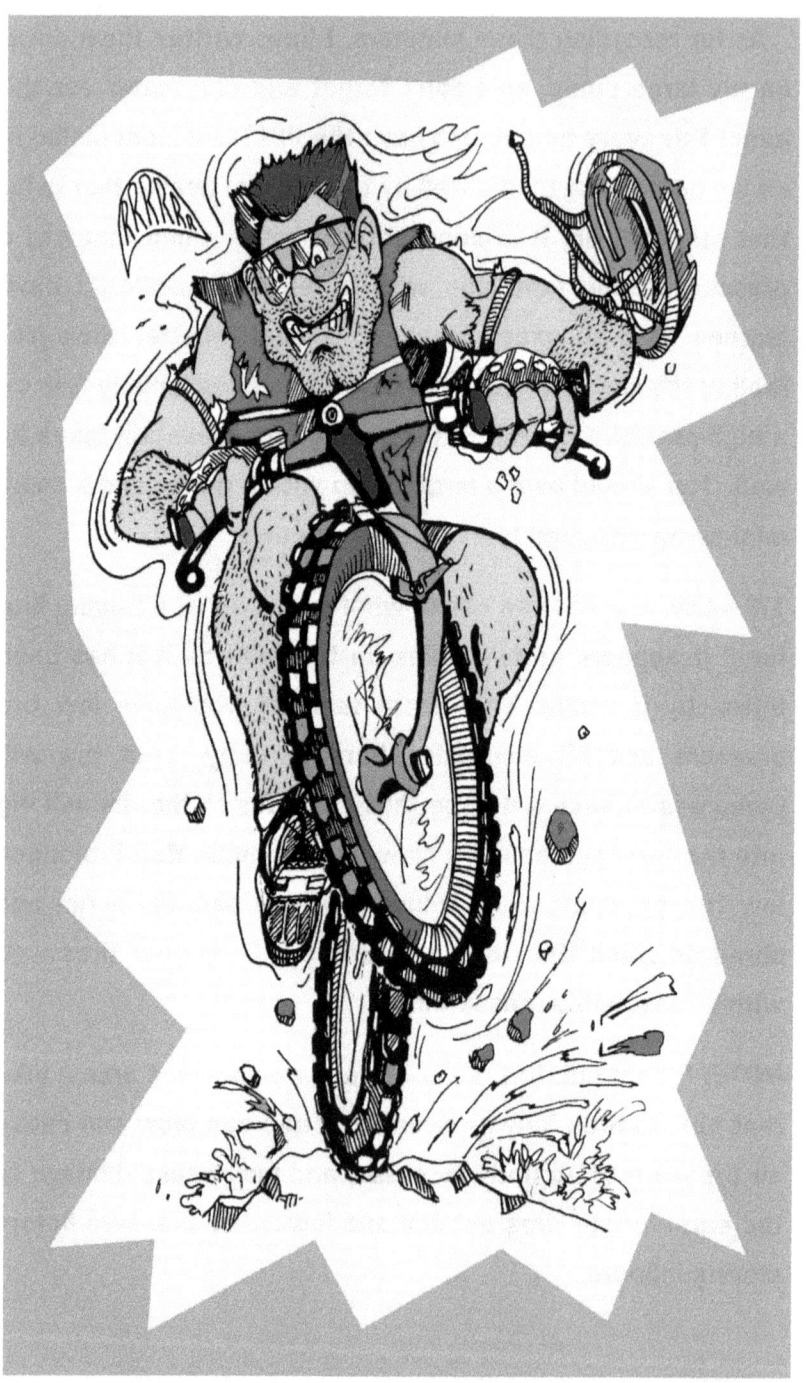

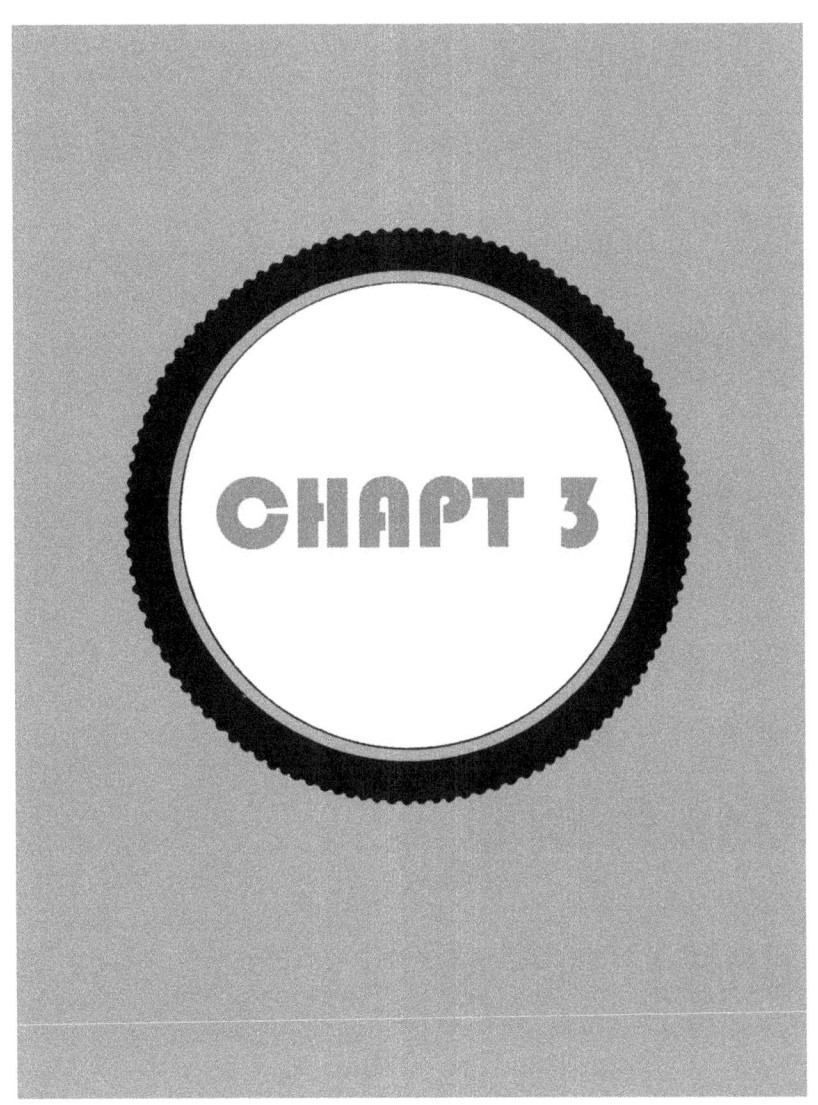

PART SMART - THE ART OF THE GAME CHANGER PARTS

BARS

STEM

SADDLES

TIRES

CHAINRINGS

GRIPS

PEDALS

BARS

Only second to the stem, handlebars are up there as one of the foremost parts that can enhance or detract from the feel of a bike in a big way. Handlebars come in a great variety of shapes, styles, lengths, and colors. There are riser bars, flat bars (no rise), moustache bars, road bike bars (drop bars), bullhorn bars, touring bars, and everything in between. A riser bar, for example, can be wide or relatively short in width. It can also have a 1-, 2-, 3- or 4-inch rise to it. And it can have a good amount of backward sweep or be almost straight in sweep. A lot of variations to the same type of bar. So, I'll stick to this type because it's the most common.

The width of handlebars can change a bike's steering dynamics. Bar size is all personal preference, and most people have their favorite width. Big bars give a big bike feel to a bike, and loose lax steering, which is desirable to some people. While narrower bars, on the other hand, give a tighter racing bike feel, and solicit an edgy steering experience. Which, too, is desirable to some.

Handlebar sweep can change your cycling attitude also. Handlebar sweep is an arching backward bend that most riser bars have. Less sweep will provoke a responsive and dirt bike feeling. More sweep, on the other hand, offers a less reactive and leisurely ride, as is the case of some urban bike bars.

The sweep of any bar can be lessened by simply rotating the bar more forward. This is called "handlebar roll." It gives a bar with a good amount of sweep a more energetic dirt bike feel. You need to do a bit of experimenting to find the right bar width, rise, sweep and roll position. Bar width, rise, sweep and roll, even in exceedingly small increments of measure, can change the handling or feel of your bike, and how you feel about biking in general, which matters!

TIP 1 – In general, a bike's handlebar width should be a little wider than the rider's shoulders. If your bars are too small, you will feel as though you can't relax. If your bars are too long, your upper body will be locked, where you can't respond well.

TIP 2 – Steel or aluminum riser bars? Steel bars smooth out bumps very well, but are a bit heavy. Aluminum bars, on the other hand, offer less in the department of deadening vibrations, but are lighter. Something to consider.

NOTE: If you are handy with a hacksaw or a pipe cutter, you can trim down handlebars if they are too wide. Remember to file down the edges.

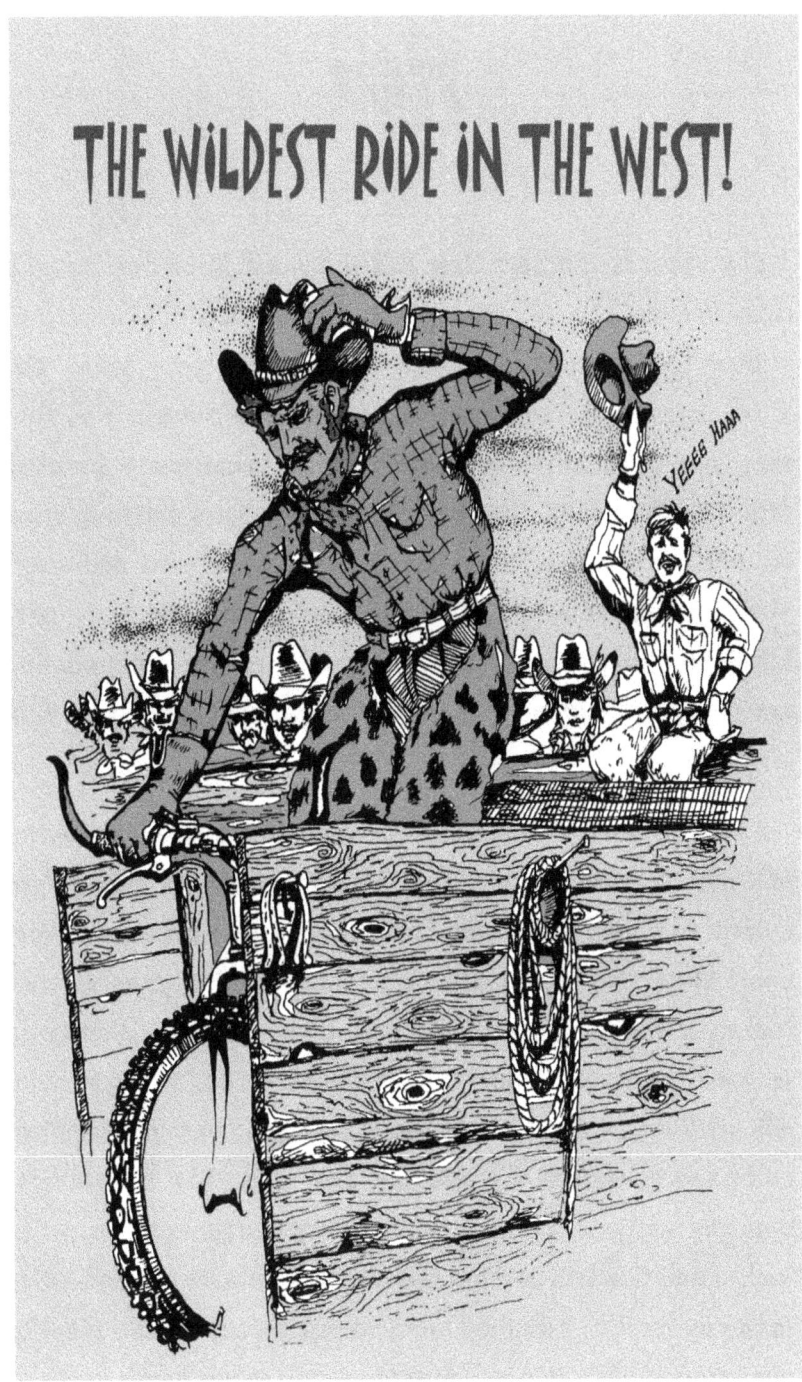

STEM

The stem is the part that has the most influence on your ride, second to none. Its length and degree of rise add or subtract considerably to the handling of your bike. The handlebars and stem need to be paired in such a way that they are considered one unit and complimentary to each other. A while back, the norm was narrow bars and long stem for mountain bikes. Now, the norm is wide bars and short stem for both mountain and hybrid bikes. Presently, the newer bikes are designed with a longer top tube. This innovation in geometry, as a whole, is designed to run a shorter stem with wide bars.

A small stem and long bars work well and offer solid control and rider positioning on mountain bikes. But, as far as light hybrid and road bikes are concerned, I feel an excessively short stem size makes steering feel too twitchy, nervy, and reactive. This is made even worse by these bikes' thin large wheels having less contact with the road. So, a longer stem will slow steering responsiveness down and put some control and ease back into the cockpit. The stem, like handlebars, requires some experimentation. Very small increments in length and rise will change the feel of your bike in more ways than you realize. You may want to buy an adjustable stem to play around with, in order to find what rise works for you.

TIP 1 – Clamp sizes differ on stems. The three main sizes are 22.2mm (steel bars), 25.4mm (standard), and 31.8mm (oversized). Make sure the stem you buy has the right clamp size for your bars.

TIP 2 – You buy a stem online and think the graphics on it are bad. In fact, they suck! You need the stem because it is the right size, but it will make your bike look goofy if you install it. What can you do? You can remove the graphics by scrubbing them off using some nail polish remover on a scrubbing sponge. It may take some elbow grease, but it will remove the graphics and make it look fine.

TIP 3 – How do you know if your stem is too short? Stand over the bike in a riding position and look down at your handlebars. If you can see your hub and wheel quick-release skewer from this position, your stem is too small. They should be blocked by your stem and bars. A stem that is too small can cause the handlebar to hit your knee while turning and cause injury. It also strains the front of the shoulders, and this will be noticeable during a ride. It can also cause hand numbness.

FRONT WHEEL CENTERING

Here's a good place to interject the topic of front wheel centering. Few things are as irritating while riding as looking down and seeing your handlebars not lined up to your front wheel. The alignment is off, and you need to fix the problem. Front wheel centering can be tricky if you are going to just eyeball the adjustment. And sometimes it always looks like the wheel is deviating off a bit left or right no matter how well you adjust it, especially if your tires are thin or your stem is short. But here are two ways that will fix it accurately. Adjusting is done on the stem by the two bolts that attach the stem to the fork steerer tube.

You will need a rubber band or tape and a straight 1x2 inch piece of wood (or a straight wooden dowel) about 14-inches (or so) in length.

First, loosen the bolt to the top cap on the fork steerer tube. Loosen only enough so that the stem can swivel somewhat freely while the top cap maintains some compression on the headset. Second, loosen the bolts on the stem that secure the stem to the fork steerer tube. Now you are ready to make the adjustment.

ADJUSTMENT FOR BIKES WITH A RIGID FORK:

Take the piece of wood and run it through the front wheel spokes and lay it flat on each fork blade (post) below the V-brakes. Mount the wood with the rubber band or tape. Make sure it is flat. Now stand over the bike and look down. Adjust the handlebars in exact parallel relation to the piece of wood. Then tighten top cap bolt and stem bolts. (Illustration 1)

ADJUSTMENT FOR BIKES WITH A FRONT SHOCK:

The previous application should work for bikes with a front shock too. But if it does not, try using the top fork crowns as your guide and point of reference. Look down at your bars and line them up parallel to the crowns. The bars should line up to the edges of the crowns. When lined up, tighten top cap bolt and stem bolts. (Illustration 2)

NOTE: Make sure there is firm, but minimal, compression to the headset. The headset should not be tightly squeezed, and the steering of the handlebars should move freely. Stem compression should not be too loose either. Loose compression will cause the fork to slightly jiggle and creak upon braking. Compression is locked in by the top cap. When tightening the stem bolts, alternate ¼ turns at a time. Top ¼ turn, then bottom ¼ turn, and repeat till tight.

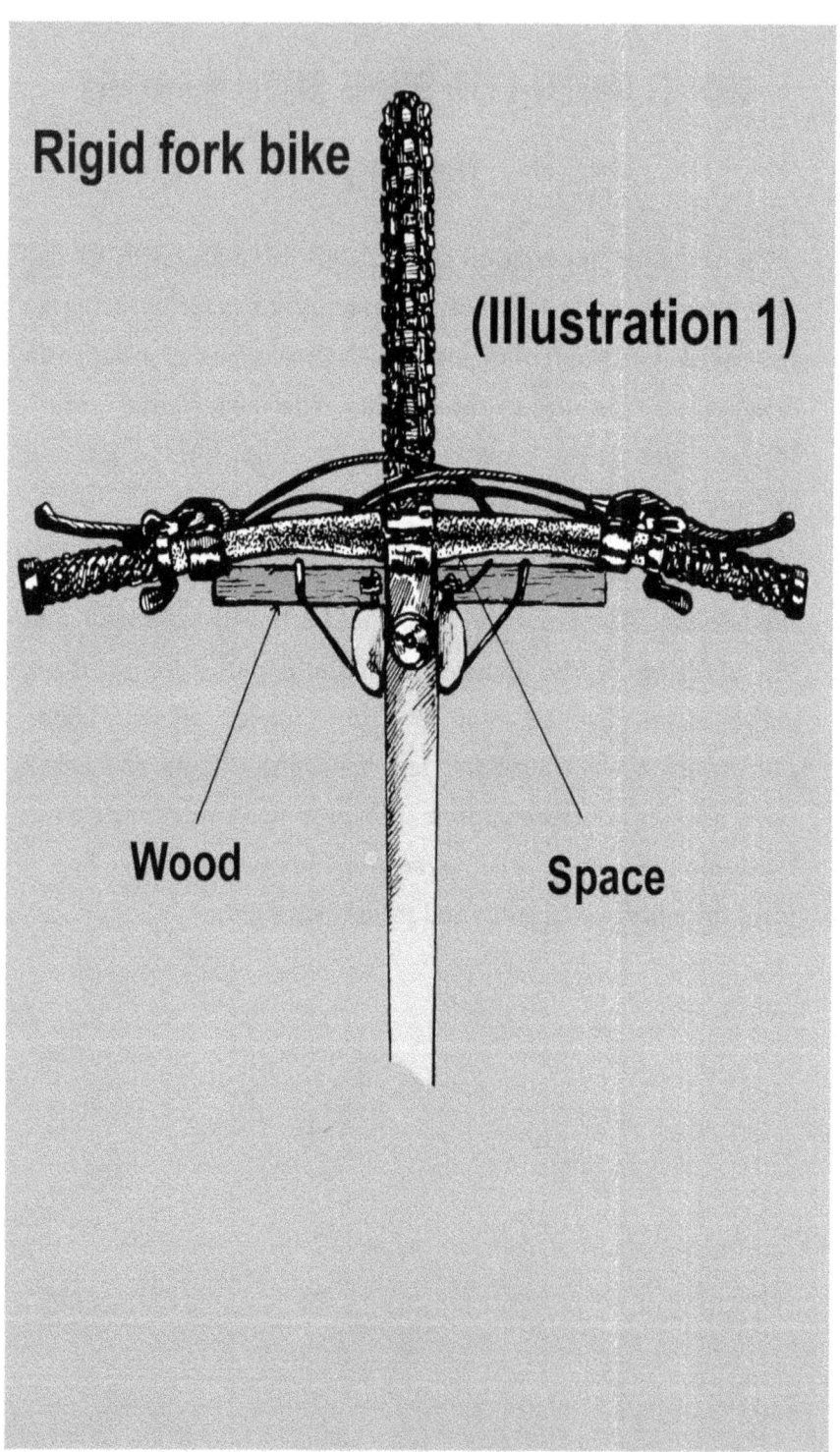

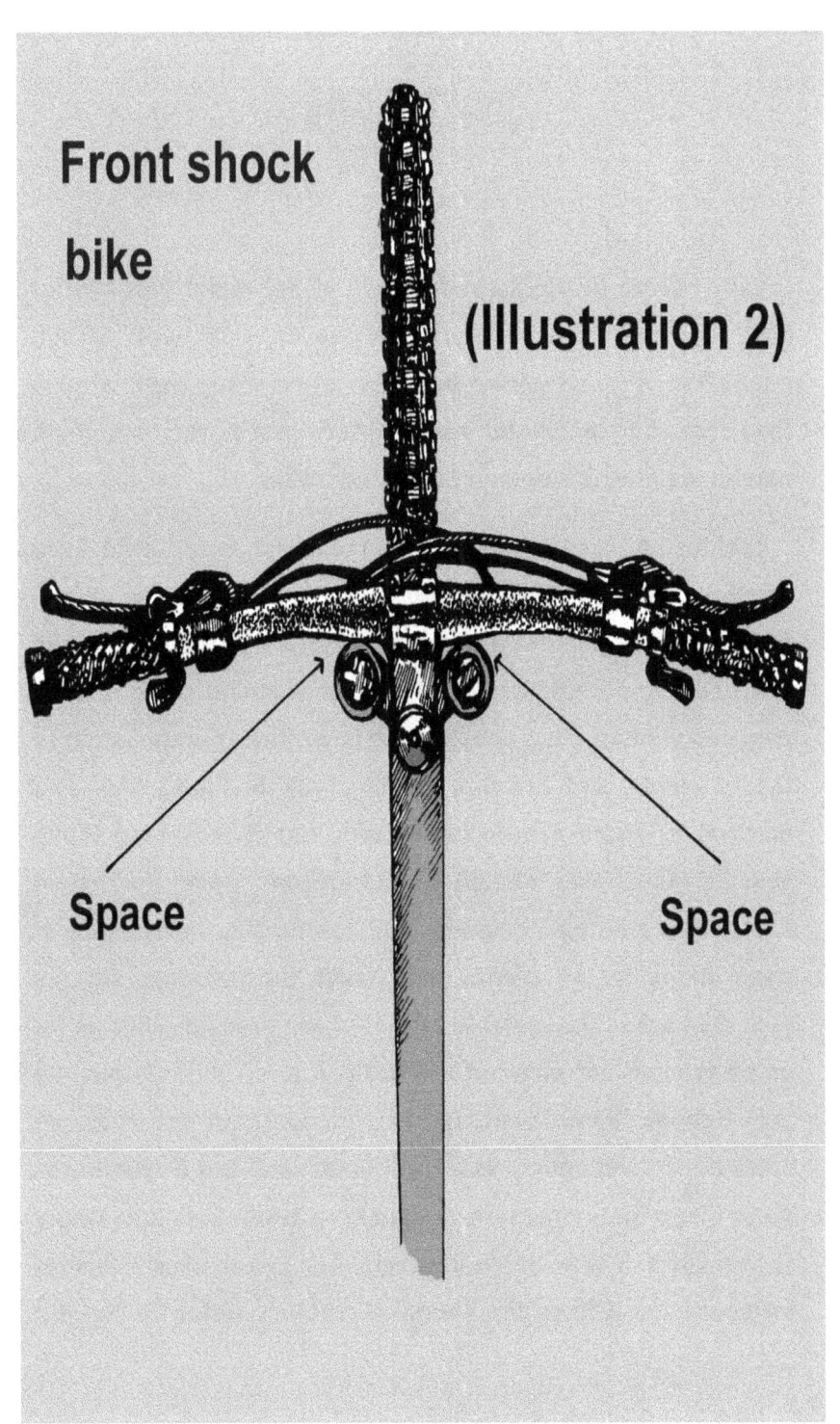

SADDLES

Your choice in a bike saddle will either make you love or hate long rides. This is something to consider well, or you might find yourself with a bad case of "monkey butt" after a long ride. And a painful and chaffed bum is not fun. Also, numbness after a ride can be considerable.

Besides the usual saddle soreness associated with hard saddles, there are medical concerns that should be noted. Saddles press against nerves and arteries that supply blood and nerve conduction to particular anatomical parts of both men and women. This constriction is verified. Compression to these nerves and arteries causes lack of blood flow and numbness. There are apprehensions about damaging these vessels, too. Bike saddle manufacturers have addressed those concerns by designing saddles that have a cavity of open space in the center that limits the pressure on this sensitive area. These seats reduce some pressure, but as far as I know, do not eliminate it 100%. I use what is known as the Hobson Easy Seat II. This seat may not look as streamlined and sporty as a traditional seat, but it eliminates all or close to all pressure to sensitive areas. It is adjustable to the width of seat bones, and it pivots. I have used this seat for years and it fixes the pressure problem perfectly. In fact,

I really love this seat and will not use any other. No "monkey butt" for me!

Given the fact that the bottom line must be met in the production of bikes, an anatomical saddle is not to be expected on any new bike, as saddles are just another part subject to the manufacturer's economical oversight. As a result, the supplied seat is very universal and basic. Which means hard and painful! So, it should be understood that in any new bike purchase, the stock saddle will have to go. You will need to go on a quest to find a new saddle, one that favors anatomical well-being and comfort. And you will have to do some homework and experimentation, too. All in all, a saddle is one of the biggest game changer parts of all.

TIP 1 – You can tilt your seat downward slightly to minimize pressure. Also, make sure your saddle is not bolted too far back on the seat rails. A saddle position that is too far back will cause you to sit on the nose of the saddle, causing numbness to one's unmentionables.

TIP 2 – The ideal saddle height should allow the rider to have a slight bend to the leg on the lowest position (the down stroke). This assures proper cadence. A saddle height that is too low will fatigue the thigh muscles. It will also make you look silly. Low saddle height is common to the beginner rider.

TIP 3 – For a comfortable ride position, the proper saddle height should ideally be lined up to the height of your handlebars. First find your perfect saddle height, then figure out which combination of riser stem height and/or riser bars height will get you to that sweet spot.

TIP 4 – Here is a good place to make mention of some instruction concerning the seatpost. The seatpost needs to have a good length of it in the frame to support the weight of the rider. As a precaution, a seatpost has an insertion marking line a few inches above the end of it. This marking line indicates the minimum length a seatpost needs to be in the frame (below the binder clamp) to support the rider's weight. Simply put, you should not be able to see this marking when your seatpost is inserted in the frame of your bike. If this line is visible, your seatpost is too high. Subsequently, any weight on it will cause the frame to bend at that point and destroy it. Your bike will only be good for spare parts. So, if you need more length to your seatpost, buy a longer one (its size is written on it next to the insertion mark). It's far better to have the insertion marking line well into the frame (below the top tube) than just below the binder clamp. Just for extra measure!

TIP 5 – When you have established the seat height that works for you, it is a good idea to mark it on your seatpost. You can lightly scratch the paint on the post with a nail by following the edge of the binder clamp. You can also use a permanent marker if your post is metallic color. Marking it will ensure that you will always find the right height if you must remove the post for any reason. And remember to add some grease to your seatpost before you put it into the frame to keep it from adhering to the frame.

(SEATPOST INSERTION MARK MUST BE INSIDE THE FRAME AND NOT VISIBLE)

INCORRECT — TOO HIGH

CORRECT — BELOW FRAME

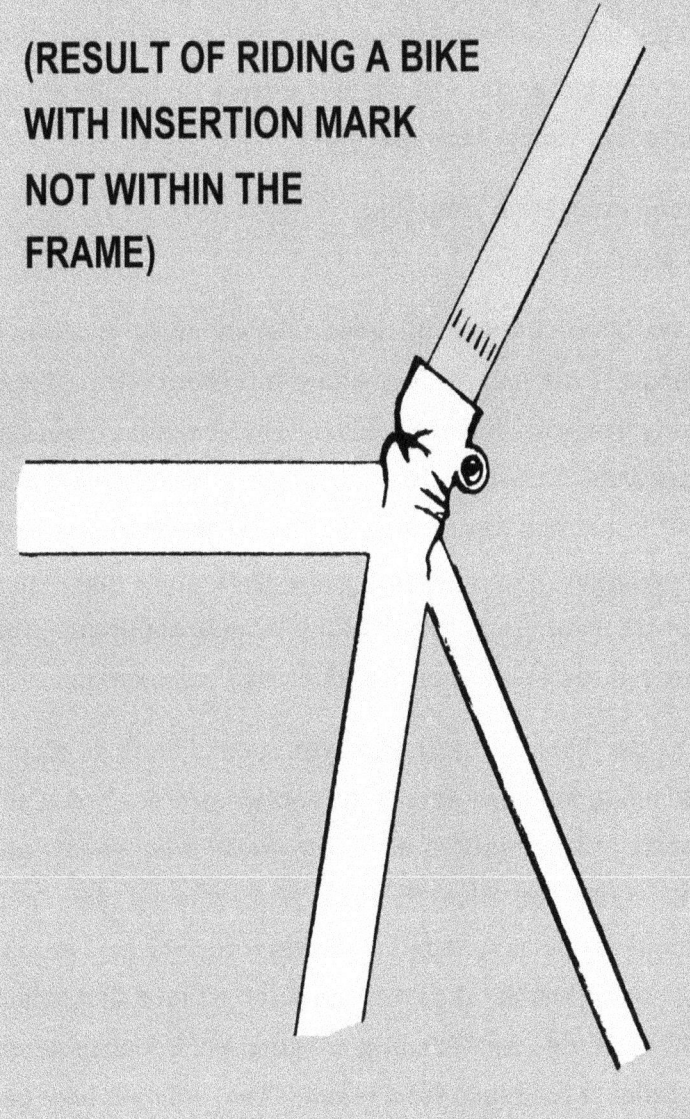

RUINED BIKE FRAME!

(RESULT OF RIDING A BIKE WITH INSERTION MARK NOT WITHIN THE FRAME)

TIRES

Tires can also greatly change the feel of your bike in big ways. Like the handlebars, stem, and saddle, tires rank high in game changer parts. And when it comes to tires, it breaks down into two simple factors:

1) Tread (knobby to smooth).
2) Tire (thick to thin).

The available mixtures of these two variables provides a wide range of choices a rider can experiment with. This is especially true with mountain bikes. Why? Because mountain bikes are built for rough riding to begin with. They have an overbuilt frame and strong wheels. So, a rider does not have to be concerned with choosing a tire that might look like it exceeds the strength capacity of the wheels and frame. This is not true of road bikes and the likes, as I will explain.

Due to the boom in new bike variations, there is also a corresponding boom in new multifunctional tires. I now see many sorts of knobby tires made for gravel bike wheels and hybrids, which can also fit road bike wheels. This new assortment in tires may tempt a new rider to deck his/her road only bike out in knobby tires and use it for gravel riding, which no doubt exceeds the bike's original purpose. Because a road bike is called a road bike for a reason. Yes, a hybrid bike can make the jump from road to gravel, being that it's dual purpose by design. But a road bike is built for the road. And this by design too. So, even though a gravel bike may look like a road bike, it is intentionally built for rough paths.

Knobby tires by nature elicit a rough riding attitude, which may spell disaster for a full-fledge road bike, if ridden accordingly. So, it's better to stay within the limitations of your bike than try to make it something it's not. To me, if you want to ride on the wild side, it's wiser to change out the bike than the tires. Besides, there are gravel specific bikes and mountain bikes to satisfy any hanker you may have for dirt.

Best advice: Switching to fatter tires is good and can add some suspension to a rigid bike. But do not go beyond the intentions of your bike; ride it for what it is.

Bottom line, when it comes to the sort of tires you're going to run on your bike, one only needs to consider the paths one is going to ride on.

TIP 1 – Plastic fenders are a good item to have as the seasons change, especially for mountain bikes, if you commute on one. They make detachable versions that can be easily put on and removed. Their price is relative to the type you buy. Remember, the bigger the tire, the wetter the backsplash on a rainy day.

TIP 2 – Tires themselves do age more rapidly if your bike is stored out in the elements. You will know this by a feeling of dullness in your tires as you ride. The springy quality of the tire now feels leathery and lifeless. Your tires can have lots of tread still left, but they're dead. Keep your bike away from the elements as best you can, and if it must be outside, cover it well. Dead tires feel like wooden wagon wheels.

TIP 3 – Inspect your tires before each ride to make sure there are no thorns or glass embedded in them. A thorn can look like any piece of road debris stuck on your tire at casual glance. Eventually any thorn or glass will work its way through the tire, puncturing the tube.

(Seating tires found in Chapter 5, **TUBES**)

NOTE: Tires have tread arrows on the sides of them. These tread arrows indicate which way a tires tread is to be facing. The tread arrows must point forward to the front of the bike.

WHEELS-RIMS

Here is a good place to interject the topic of rims. Rims don't usually give you any problems if you are a moderate rider and have double wall rims. But if you have single wall rims, you do have to ride with some caution to avoid the big hits, and as a result, a bent rim. A bent rim is no fun and necessitates truing. Proper wheel truing requires a truing stand and finesse, not to mention patience. It is a matter of tightening and loosening spokes in order to achieve proper wheel roundness (radial trueness) and rim straightness (lateral trueness). This is an art, and the big jobs are best left to those who have the knowledge, experience and tools to deal with it. To the novice, a bent rim would certainly be outside his/her range of skill, maybe to the average rider as well. Fixing attempts come with the potential to make things worse. So, best not goof with it unless you know exactly what you're doing. I would just take it to a bike shop if the job is a big one. And if the price of repair is too high, measure it up against the price of a new wheel. It may be cheaper to just buy a new wheel. You can also search for some hole in the wall bike repair shop. Sometimes good deals and highly-experienced people can be found where you least expect them. Have an open mind!

Broken spokes should always be replaced promptly. And most riders can easily do it, assuming you can remove a cassette or freewheel, if it's the back wheel. You should never ride a bike with a missing spoke or spokes.

TIP 1 – While riding hard and taking a big hit or even dismounting improperly, a wheel can sustain a large warping of the rim. This great distortion is called a "taco'd rim." This is different from that of a simple bent rim in that the warping is throughout the entire wheel. Your wheel looks like a "potato chip." A "taco'd rim" can be forced back into its shape with the weight of the rider by removing the wheel, then standing on the rim and jumping lightly on the high points. You can also leverage it against a 2x4 or against a tree. You can also strike it to the ground. You can fine tune it with a spoke wrench after it gets close to straight. It took a blunt force to create the warping and takes blunt force to fix it. But it must be done right. It's an all or nothing proposition because it might not work. And use it as a last resort to avoid a long walk.

TIP 2 – Extra emergency spokes can be stored on your bike by taping them to the chainstay opposite of the cogs.

TIP 3 – All spokes should be checked from time to time for looseness. Spoke looseness can be checked by plucking them like a harp string. A loose spoke will sound dull and different than those with proper tension. It will also feel like it has less tension. It must be tightened. Also make sure that the spoke tool you use is the right size for the spoke nipples of your rims. If it is even slightly bigger than your spoke nipples, it will strip them. If your spoke nipples squeal as you turn them, they will each need to be oiled with a drop of oil.

NOTE: Every rider should beef up his/her knowledge of basic wheel truing. Learning how to use a truing stand and spoke wrench can be gratifying and empowering. An understanding of spokes and how they work will keep you out of the dark and from being under the mercy of those who practice this pricey mystical art.

CHAINRINGS

On most low to mid-end bikes, you will have a crankset consisting of aluminum cranks and a set of steel chainrings. These chainrings themselves cannot be replaced or changed out like higher end bikes, because they are permanently attached to one crank and are riveted together. This creates a dilemma if you do not like their size ratio. You must buy a totally new crankset if you want to change them out, which equates to big money as far as parts are concerned.

Now as I said earlier, most mountain bikes, and this is starting to be true of some hybrids, are now being sold today (in both bike stores and department stores) with a set of skimpy toothed triple chainrings consisting of a tooth number of 42/34/24 (which means tiny chainrings!) and similar ratios. Not the usual 48/38/28 or similar combination. Essentially, this new gearing is for hill riding and not for the road as the older ratio was. For obvious reasons, a cheap low-end mountain bike lookalike is not a true mountain bike. It is simply not built for that kind of abuse. Sometimes it will even say on its label that it is not intended for mountain riding. So why do the manufacturers insist on gearing it for the hills? Better to gear it for the road, since they know that is all it can handle. And a fitness hybrid is certainly not a trail bike. So why gear it as a trail bike? It's a road bike! Go figure! One thing is for sure, this factor can add an unnecessary hitch to buying your bike, because cranks should not have to be swapped out straight-off-the-bat. So, the importance of this topic cannot be skimmed over.

I do not understand the logic of bike manufacturers here. "What are they thinking?" Is it just another scheme to save money? Or to set a speed limit on bikes? I don't know. These chainrings will never give you the needed speed to ride in the streets happily. And I don't see how this gearing will go unnoticed to a rider. As you ride, you will keep saying, "Where's the speed I used to have?" and spin your cranks in utter frustration.

So, this is something to think about. They will have to be changed out if you do road riding. And you will probably need some help in ordering because there are some specific details to ordering cranksets, like crank length and bottom bracket axle compatibility. This can be done with relative ease if you buy from a bike shop. The pain of having to change out your cranks early on adds a totally unnecessary additional cost to your purchase, which is substantial. In addition to the added cost of a new set of cranks, it is likely (not always) that you will have to change out your freewheel or cassette, too. Why? Because there might be cog ratios on your bike that favor hill riding as well. You will also need a new chain, or may have to add links to your chain for more length. I don't mean to scare you away. In fact, it might not even matter to you. Or you might favor these new chainring sizes, being that you may live in hill country.

TIP 1 – Chainrings can be cleaned using a discarded dish brush or an old toothbrush.

TIP 2 – Occasionally take hold of a crankarm and push and pull on it laterally from side to side, to see if there is any play. There should not be any. If there is, check the fixing bolts on both sides (check the fixing bolts regularly). If they are tight, check the retainer cup (for sealed cartridge type). Tighten if loose with a cartridge retainer ring tool. You will have to remove the left crankarm for that.

TIP 3 – When ordering a new crankset, make sure that you order the right crankarm size.

TIP 4 – Never grease the end of the axle that goes into the crankarm. This needs to be dry to prevent the crankarm from sliding too deep while torquing and cracking the crankarm.

TIP 5 – When buying a new bike, inspect for wear or paint missing on the chainrings. Wear or bare metal on black painted chainrings is a telltale sign that the bike was used and might have been returned. Dirty tires are also an indicator of a returned bike.

NOTE: There is a term for the smallest chainring on a set of three chainrings (triple-ring crankset). It is called the "Granny Gear." The "Granny Gear" is used to go uphill and in the steepest of inclines. Use it with the largest rear cog on a steep ascend.

Quick reference guide for beginners on chainring/cog combinations. For:

SPEED RIDING: Use big chainring and smallest cog.

MODERATE UPHILL RIDING: Use middle chainring and middle cog.

EXTREME UPHILL RIDING: Use small chainring and large cog.

Gears to the right are for speed. Gears to the left are for uphill.

Learn to analyze different bikes and ask questions to other riders. Questions like how certain parts or item positions work for them? What do they bring along on their rides? Be inquisitive! Also, look into innovations that will improve your riding experience. Bikes and gadgets are always evolving. Then do some experimentation. Always keep learning ways to better your ride!

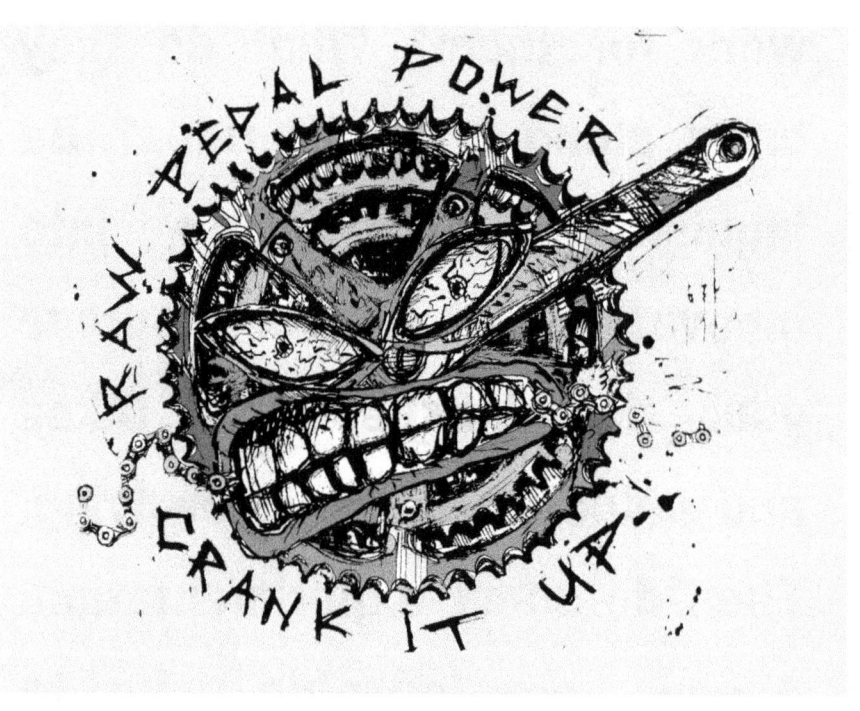

GRIPS

Grips don't make or break a bike, but they do go a long way in the feel and look of your bike, as well as function. A while back, and not too far, most bikes that were sold had grips that would mimic the rugged chunky pattern of knobby tires. This was especially true for mountain bikes. It looked cool! But today, most bikes are sold with smoother and thinner grips, including mountain bikes. Is this because there is a big slant to minimalism these days, and bikes are just reflecting this trending fashion? Possibly. Or is it just simply company cheapness? Some may see this style as a negative, an emasculation of the hardy grip. But I see it as bicycle grip evolution.

ASSUMPTION

One assumes that thick is always better, because obviously, the more rubber between the hand and bar, the better the grasp. One also assumes that the more texture on a grip, the better the grasp. And that more rubber and texture take care of the numbness issue too. But here are my thoughts on the matter from my experience:

LOGICAL DEDUCTION

Grip thickness: The thicker the grip, the less one's fingers can wrap tightly around it, meaning a weaker grasp. As a result, the rider grasps even harder, producing strain and fatigue in the hands, and an even weaker grasp. Thicker is not better!

Grip texture: The more textured the grip, the more open spaces in between, creating less palm contact. Less palm contact means reduced grasp. More texture is not better!

So, even though a leaner, less textured grip is not exactly burly or cool looking, it offers more grasping power, superior to thicker. And beyond logical deduction, I find this to be true through trial and error. Here, less can be more! And what works for tires does not necessarily work for grips. Makes sense! But what about hand numbness?

IN MATTERS CONCERNING HAND NUMBNESS, HERE ARE SOME AREAS TO LOOK INTO:

1) **Grip density** (hard grips hurt).
2) **Stem height and length** (wrong combinations can put more weight on the palms).
3) **Handlebar height** (low bars can put more weight on the palms).
4) **Lack of gloves or using the wrong type of gloves** (means no padding on key areas).
5) **Saddle positioning** (a saddle that is too far back causes the rider to ride on the saddle nose. The rider compensating to this uncomfortable position puts more weight on the hands. Thus, numbness!).

PLATFORM GRIPS

Somewhat new to the grip market are comfort grips. Comfort grips have a "platform" or "wings" for the palms of your hands to rest on. They offer a medium grip thickness and a flat broad area to rest the palms of one's hands. These are a good innovation. But they are not that good on the downhill. Reason being, the "wings" become an obstacle to the hand for getting a good grip, as your hand position changes going downhill. You end up having to grasp over the wing which is now in the center of your hand. But they certainly offer welcomed comfort on a flat and long ride. Personally, I use only the softer and thinner types. I find the harder and thicker types to actually contribute to numbness.

The takeaway: Experiment and find out what works best for you. The choices in grips are almost infinite, and so are the stem and handlebar combinations. Remember, a stem and handlebar combination that works for someone else may not work for you. The same with grips. Everyone's body is different, and hand sizes are also a big factor.

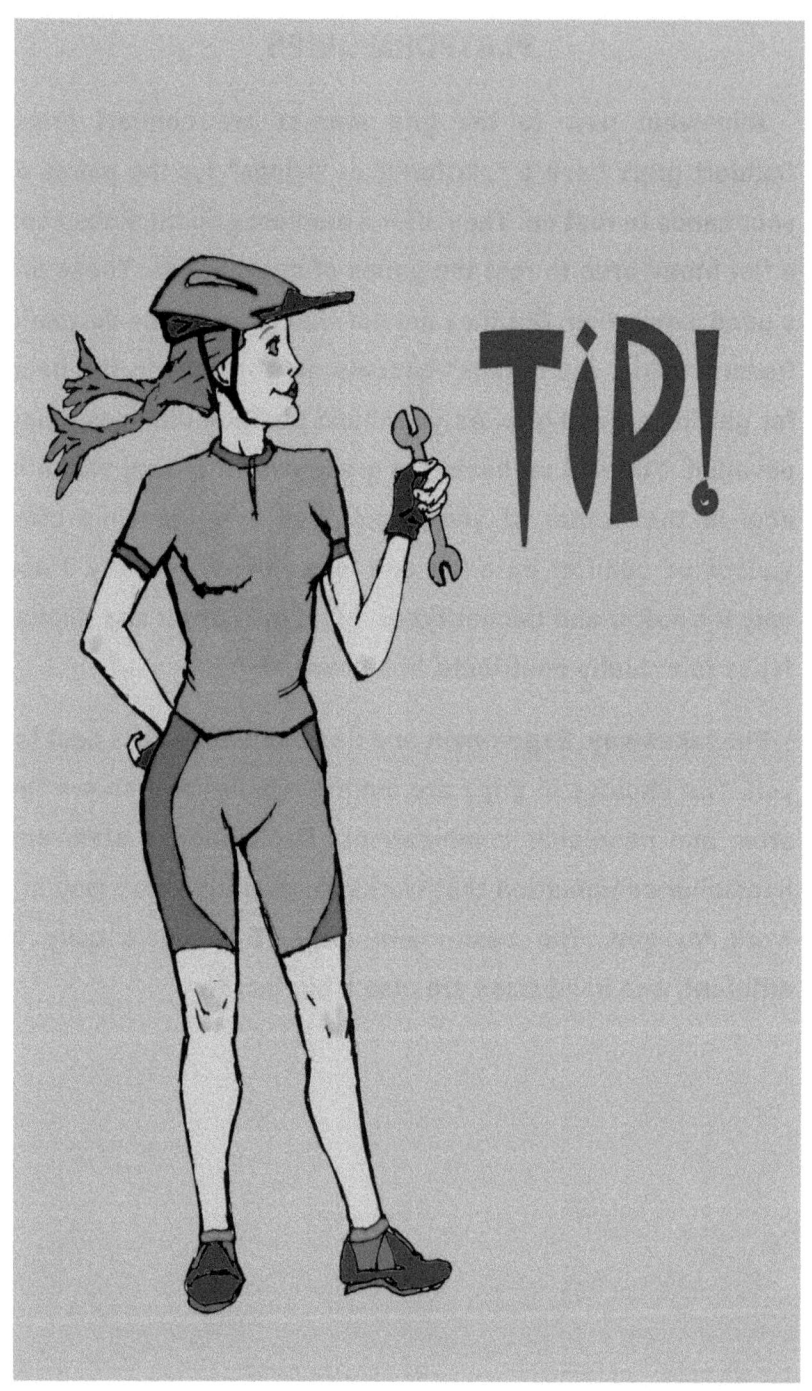

TIP 1 – To remove grips, I usually run a thin piece of wood (usually the handle of a thin paintbrush or chopstick) between the grip and handlebars and slide it in as far as I can. Then I position the bars at a slant so that gravity will assist as I squirt some water or hair spray in. I wiggle the chopstick, then remove it. After that, I just twist and pull the grip off. If you have an air compressor, you can blow air between the grip and handlebar and slide the grip off. Do not use a cutter blade to remove grips. It will scratch into your handlebars.

New grips can be installed after you clean the bars. Apply some alcohol to the inside of the new grips and on the surface of the bars, and slide the new grips in place. Wait about a day to ride, so the alcohol can dry. You can also use hair spray. If you are going to ride immediately, just lightly moisten the bar with water and hit the grip in place with the palm of your hand.

TIP 2 – There are many uses for old grips, such as making chainstay protectors out of them or using them on your bar ends. You can also use pieces of them between the mounts and handlebars for any lights you attach to your bike.

NOTE 1: Save the grips that still have some life in them. Grips are expensive!

NOTE 2: Silicone grips are now used by most pro mountain bikers. I use them and highly recommend them.

PEDALS

Obviously, all bikes come with pedals, but these parts, too, are usually changed and customized early on. Why? Because most serious riders need to have some form of locking mechanism that secures their shoes to the pedal, allowing better cadence and power. Pedals alone are not adequate because they come with no such device. Nor do they usually have features to accommodate (on cheap pedals) the bolts and straps for basic toeclips, if you would like to install some. So, an upgrade is necessary, and there are choices to make as to what type of locking apparatus is needed.

CLIPLESS PEDALS VS. TOECLIPS AND STRAPS

Unless you are a serious sport rider, I do not see the need for expensive clipless pedals. With clipless pedals you need to buy special shoes. A lot of these shoes limit your ability to walk if your bike fails in some way, because they are simply not walking shoes. I do understand these shoes help in your performance as you ride, because they have a rigid sole and are designed for riding. But to me, they just seem overdressed, overpriced, and not practical at all.

My vote is for composite plastic pedals with plastic toeclips and straps. I do realize these are old school, but they are far more user-friendly. Why plastic pedals and plastic toeclips?

Metal pedals and metal toeclips can cut into your shin very deeply if your shin hits them, which happens a lot. I personally have had that experience. Many riders have scars on their shins for this reason. Plastic will cause less damage. A gashed shin can end a ride quickly.

Toeclips and straps are getting harder to find. I went to one bike shop and asked for them, and the sales staff did not know what I was talking about. After explaining, they looked at me as though I was asking for some bike relic accessory from the ancient past.

Toeclips and strapless toe clips (a variation of toeclip that does not use straps) come in different sizes, small, medium and large. Both types will allow you to get off your bike and explore, because they can be used with any shoe.

Both clipless and toeclips and straps type pedals, allow the rider to pull up on the pedals and employ different muscles. This gives an advantage over just pedals alone, because you can utilize muscles that are not fatigued.

TIP 1 – You may have to drill holes in the plastic pedals if they do not have any, to install the toeclips. Make sure the pedals are structurally enforced enough to handle the holes.

TIP 2 – On the threaded axle bolt of each pedal, there is an imprinted "R" or "L" at the end. These stand for "left" and "right." By these markings you will know which pedal is the right one for the crankarm in relation to you in standing position on your bike. Pedals should be screwed in by hand

and then tightened with a wrench. If it is hard to screw in or is not screwing in, do not force it. Consider whether you are tightening it straight. If it is not tightened straight, forcing it will ruin the threading on the crankarm.

NOTE 1: You should be able to pull your shoe out of your toeclips with ease as you dismount your bike. If there is even a bit of difficulty pulling your shoe out, your toeclip straps are too tight. You don't want your shoes to get locked in even slightly. Any delay in getting your shoe out will cause you to fall over as you dismount your bike. So, keep your straps reasonably snug, not too tight, or too loose.

NOTE 2: A good thing to remember when removing pedals and trying to figure out the direction of the threading is this: Looking down at your bike (facing forward), you should turn the pedal wrench (from upward position) to the direction of the rear of the bike to unscrew. This is the same for both pedals. And opposite to tighten. Pedal threading is meant to tighten as you pedal by forward motion.

NOTE 3: Strapless toeclips will not allow a rider to pull up on the pedal while riding. This is disappointing. So, remember this before buying. But they will allow a rider to have that locked-in feel and will keep the rider's shoes in place.

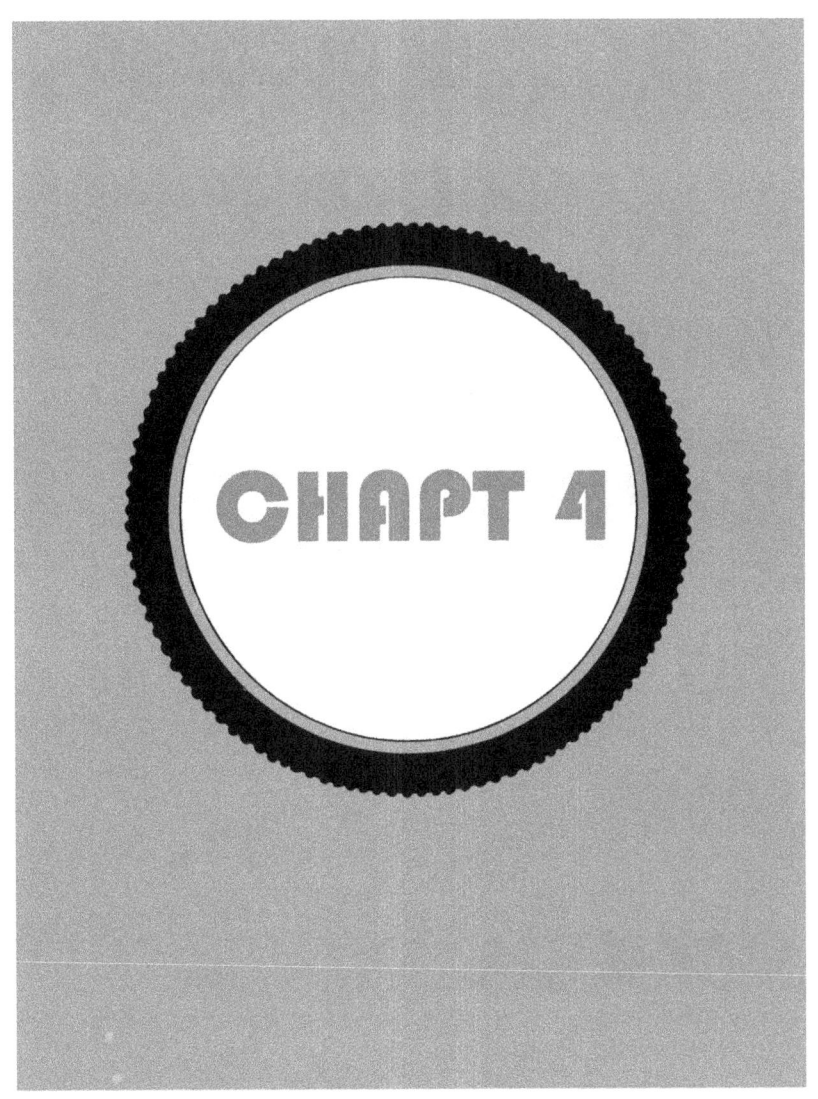

ACCESSORY SMART - THE ART OF CHOOSING ACCESSORIES

LIGHTS

KICKSTAND

MINI PUMP

RACK

SADDLE BAG

WATER BOTTLE AND CAGES

BAR ENDS

BELL

COMPUTER

MIRROR

TIRE LINERS

CONSIDER THIS:

Department store accessories are becoming better and better. The quality and the designs, to me, are, with a few exceptions, just as high-quality as if you purchase them from a bike store. Many brands are of excellent quality and reasonably priced. They last just as long, too. Given the rough nature of cycling, they should not be expected to last forever anyway. So, either way, bike store bought, or department store bought, you'll have to replace them every few years.

I think it is nonsense to hold the opinion that you must buy your accessories from a bike store to be a legitimate cyclist. Many cycle elitists look down on riders who buy their accessories at department stores. To some elitists, these people are "cheap." Yes, a bike should be purchased at a bike store if you can. But I see no need to waste money buying accessories at a bike store. That being said, I do think that the local bike store should be supported.

LIGHTS

Your bike must have a headlight and rear light if you are going to ride in the dark. A steady white front light and a steady or flashing rear red light. With the advent of LED lights, there is now a plethora of powerful and reasonably priced light sets to choose from. These light sets use small batteries and can operate a very long time before new batteries are needed. In my opinion, the most useful front lights are those that consist of a plastic/aluminum flashlight fastened to the handlebars via its plastic mounting device. If an occasion occurs where you need a portable hand-held light quickly, you simply unscrew the retainer screw and slide the light out. When you are done, slide it back in and retighten the retainer screw.

In addition to the main headlight and rear, I think it is prudent to have a pair of weaker flashing lights—a white flashing light for the front (secondary to main steady light) and a red flashing light for the rear (secondary to rear steady light). This is good for your basic city night riding, since you need a strong headlight to see, and flashers to be seen. Peak safety depends on optimal visibility. These can be purchased at your local department store.

If you do a lot of night wilderness and hill riding, I suggest buying a light that has some real power, whether purchased at a bike shop or online. Night hill riding requires strong lighting, both to the direct front and to the peripherals. A department store light will not do the trick.

TIP 1 – If you are not going to use your bike lights for an extended amount of time, do this: Remove your front and back lights and remove the batteries. Tie a rubber band around the batteries so the contact points do not touch each other. Get two resealable zip-lock plastic bags and store both the lights and the batteries inside separately till needed. Batteries left unused and unchecked inside any electric device for an extended time will leak and corrode, destroying the inner metal parts. So, separate the batteries, and protect your lights.

Many bike lights now being sold are charged via USB port. Yes, no batteries to deal with! I find this very convenient and practical. So, consider this in choosing a light set.

TIP 2 – Before purchasing any front light, **MAKE SURE** the mounting clamp of the light can accommodate the **THICKNESS** of your bars. Your bars will be one of three:

- Thin type, 22.2mm (steel bars).
- Medium type, 25.4mm (standard).
- Thick type, 31.8mm (oversized).

TIP 3 – When you mount your rear light (to the seatpost), make sure it clears the height of your rear tire. Otherwise, the rear tire can block the light from those who need to see it (those who are behind the rider). Having a saddle bag may also lower the rear light too far, especially if you have a small size bike. Be aware of this and make sure it's visible.

NOTE: Night riding lights do not take the place of reflectors. Reflectors are still needed and should not be removed from a bike. You should check your city and state laws concerning bicycle lights and reflectors for legal requirements.

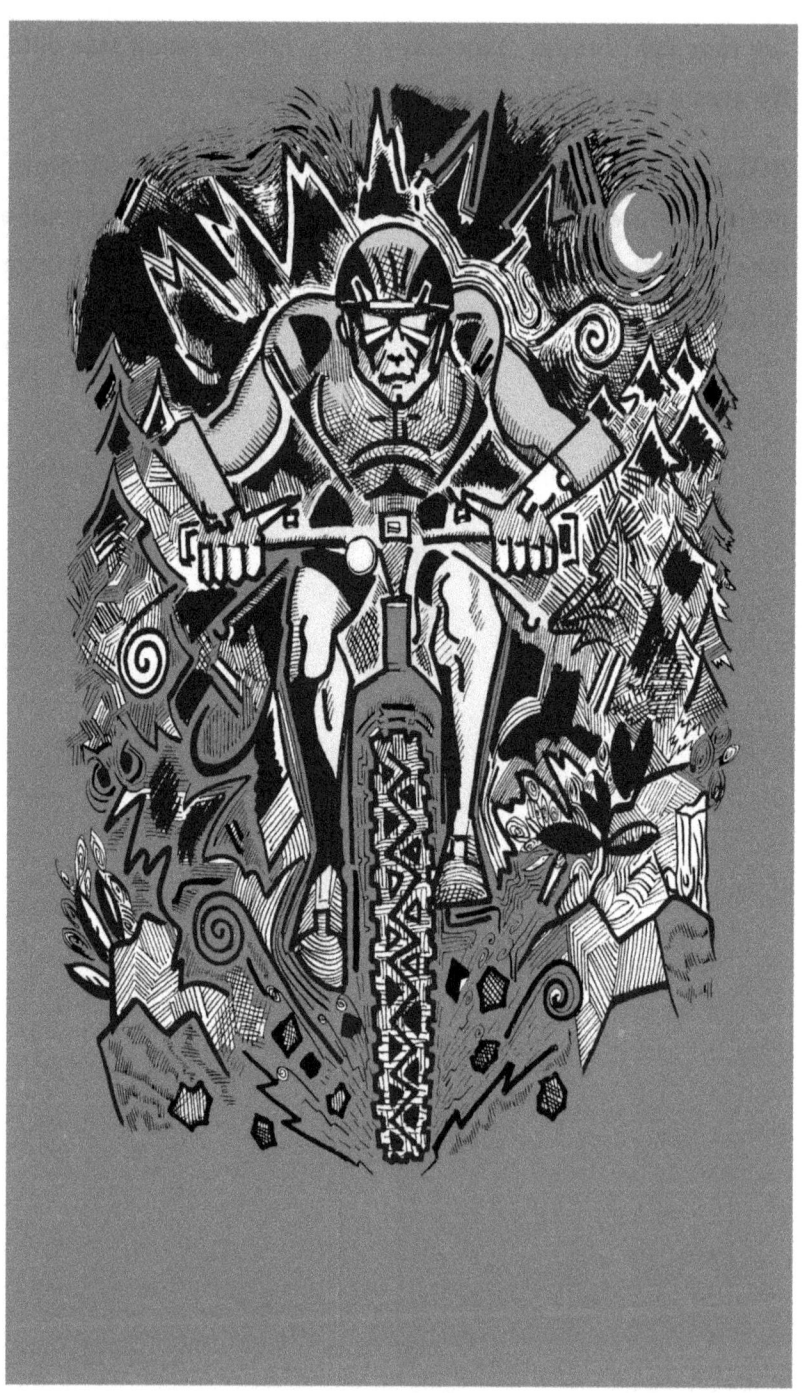

KICKSTAND

Kickstand, should I, or shouldn't I? To me, a kickstand is a must. It weighs practically nothing, and doesn't get in the way of pedaling too much. There is not always a place to rest a bike upright, and without a kickstand you are left with one option, to lay it down on the dirt or pavement. Letting your bike rest on the dirt or pavement is not good for your bike, and someone can trip on it. It ruins the grips and scratches up the saddle and pedals. Plus, even a leaning bike propped against something seems to always slide from its position and fall over on something. It usually ends up getting its finish and graphics scratched up in the process.

When it comes to kickstands, there are two main styles to choose from. The most often used kickstand (standard) is the one that is bolted to the frame near the cranks. The second style is mounted further back to the seatstay and chainstay, via clamp. Another version of the second type is one that is mounted only to the chainstay with bolts (mounting holes already built into the frame). I prefer this style because it's more out of the way.

TIP – A trick of the trade on a standard kickstand: If it seems too long, do not cut it. Instead, push down (gently) against it (at center) with the bottom of your shoe sole and slightly bend it. This is easily done and will fix the problem. Be careful not to crack it by bending it too far.

MINI PUMP

The mini pump is an absolute necessity in bike riding. It's foolish to ride without one. A good pump should have both Schrader and Presta valve capabilities. If you have high pressure tires, make sure the pump you buy can pump at that PSI. I recommend testing any newly bought pump several times before you mount it on your bike and ride.

One time, I purchased an inexpensive bike pump from a local department store, mounted it, and went for a ride. I never really tested it beforehand, but assumed it worked fine. Many miles into the ride I noticed I needed some air in my front tire. I stopped and proceeded to fill the tire. But I found it was difficult to tighten the pump nozzle on the tube valve. It would not pass air into it.

So, I did what any intelligent person would do, (LOL) force it in! Then, the pump nozzle locked on the tube valve, and I could not detach it. As I pulled on it in frustration, the whole tube valve ripped right off. I was not carrying a spare tube with me that day. Needless to say, it was an awfully long walk home on a hot day.

A rare failing to a mini pump is the lever. Sometimes it can break, but not often. So, study its design before buying it. Make sure it looks sturdy. Also, avoid buying strange off-brands and pumps with many moving parts, or one that has a so-called innovative design. Keep it simple.

DO NOT buy a mini pump that has a hose (they still make them), whether it is a detachable or permanent one. A hose on a mini pump is very outdated and not necessary. It is a part that is obsolete in modern pump design. Consider it a weak point. It just adds to things that can go wrong and extra work. Here are some solid reasons to forgo this type:

1) Rubber ages and quickly deteriorates, causing hoses to crack. Cracking usually occurs at either end of the hose at the connectors. Deterioration is rarely visible and only shows itself by ripping when you create a twisting motion to the hose, like when you connect the hose to the pump when you have a flat! So, this is definitely not reliable.

2) Detachable hoses get lost while riding. And a pump without a hose is useless.

3) The hose ends need to be twist screwed to the pump and to the tube valve, adding difficulty. This is not only outdated and crude, but unnecessary, because pumps have levers now and have had them for some time. And you lose most of the air you just pumped in as you try to twist the head quickly off the tube valve. **JUST FORGET THIS TYPE OF PUMP.** Don't go backwards!

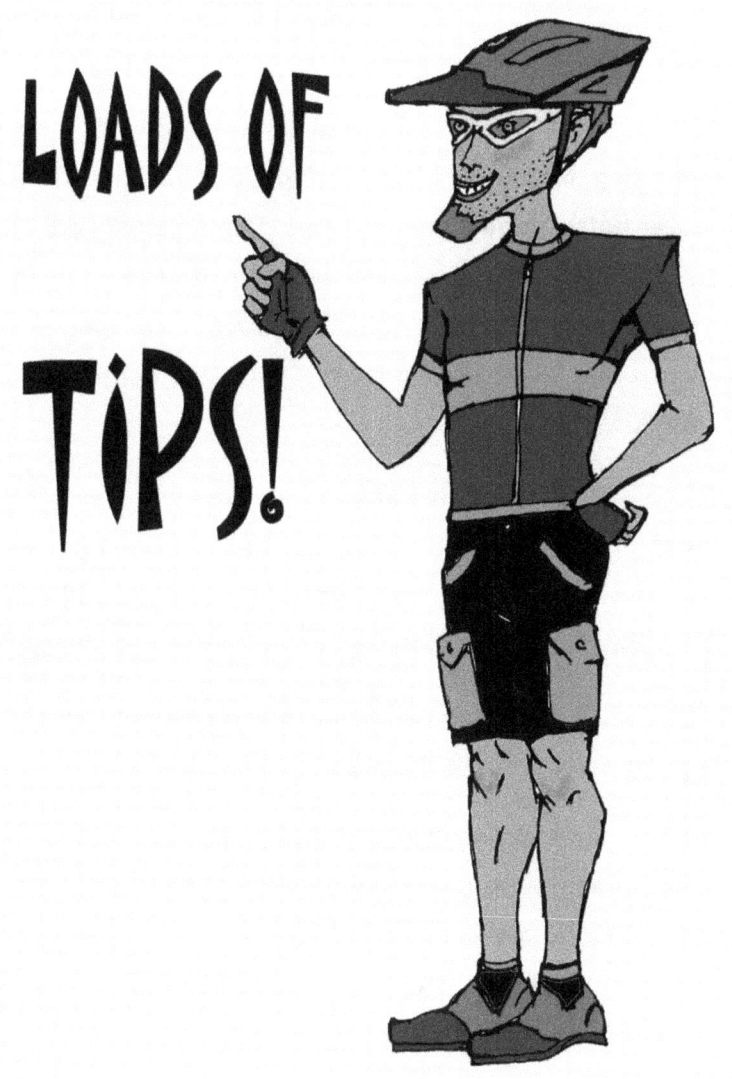

TIP 1 – Buy only well-known brands and try to stay in the middle to the highest quality model. Also, a PSI gauge would be great. Make sure (I say again) it has the least number of moving parts on it and can handle high PSI too. And again, no hoses! Bottom line: A broken pump or no pump means you walk home in the event of a flat.

TIP 2 – Most, if not all, mini pumps sold will come with mounting brackets. These attach to the same bolts your water bottle cage is mounted on. These usually come with a nylon Velcro strap to secure the pump so it will not slip out of the brackets on a hard ride. Make sure it has one. If not, buy one. A lost pump means (again) you walk home in the event of a flat.

TIP 3 – When attaching your pump to the brackets, face the front of the pump (the part that has the inlet for the tube valve) away from the front tire. Let it face the rider instead. This way no road crud flying off the tire will get inside of it.

TIP 4 – CO_2 cartridge pumps create waste and run out of air, a pointless device to the average cyclist.

NOTE: I've seen guys riding their bike with a large garage pump (hanging hose included) tied to the rear rack of their bike. Also, in a backpack as they ride. This, no doubt looks really lame. Please, just buy a normal mini pump. Mini pumps are not that expensive.

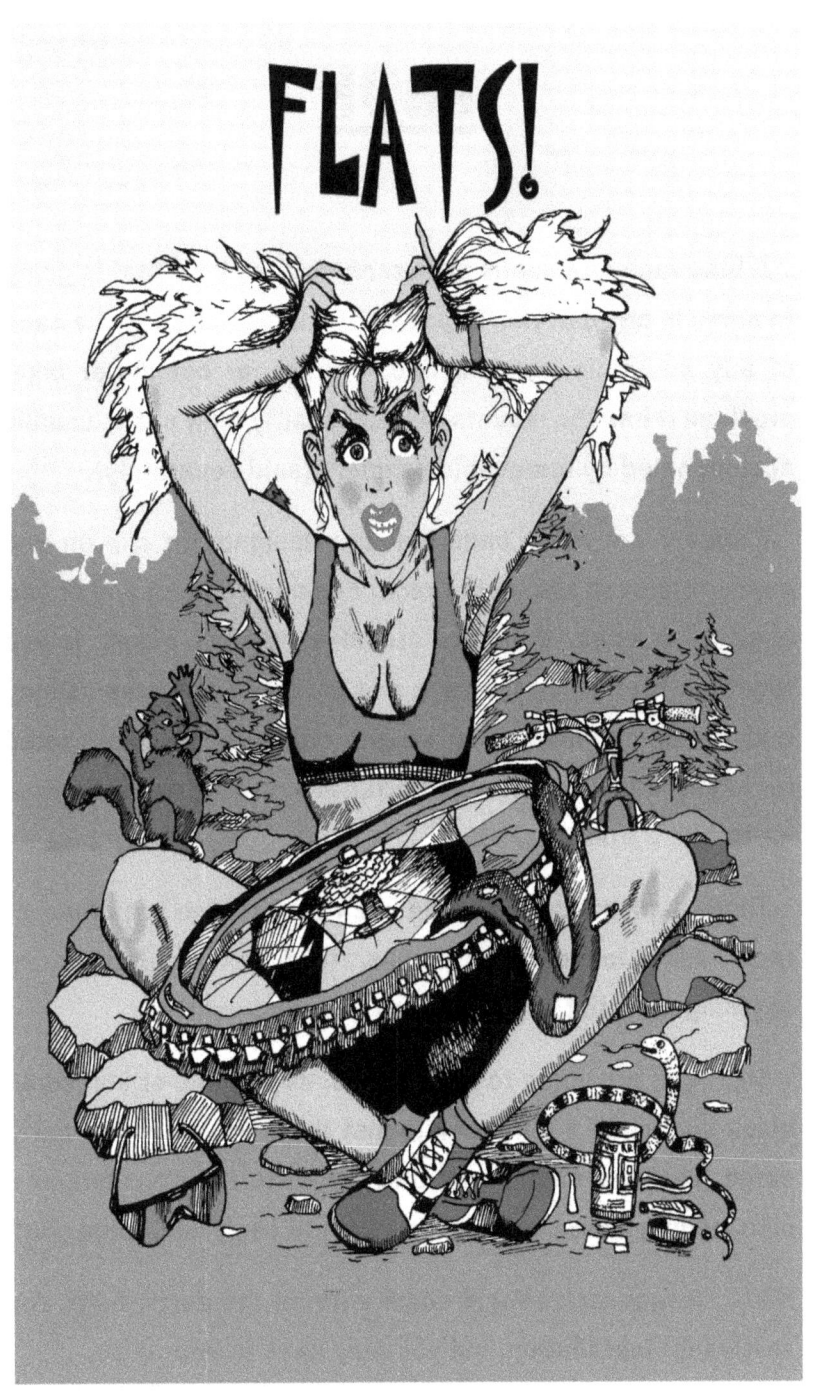

RACK

A bike rack is a useful accessory for any bike that is going to serve in any carrying capacity. It can be bolted to the back of any mountain, road, hybrid, cruiser, or commuter bike, provided it has the mounts. A rack is fairly light and is usually accompanied by removable panniers (sold separately).

Panniers are nylon bags that are designed to clip on and connect to each side of the rack. You can connect one or two bags as needed. Panniers are also sold as a set, joined together, that sit on the rack and balance each other. Being that a rack can hold much weight, panniers are constructed for heavy loads and are also better at keeping things dry than if you had a front basket.

There is also a single cargo pack that sits on top of a rear rack, used for carrying books, food, extra clothing, or anything a cyclist might need on an extended ride.

So, if you are going to run errands, do touring, or just some quick shopping, a bike rack is just the item needed to carry cargo. They do make racks that mount to the front fork of a bike, adding more capacity for a rider to carry additional stuff.

NOTE: A rear rack should come with all the parts, bolts and screws for installation, but you may have to improvise.

SADDLE BAG

A saddle bag or a wedge bag is a common accessory for most riders. It is a small, zippered nylon bag that is mounted under the saddle. Its position under the seat is out of the way and does not create any interference while riding. A saddle bag is good for carrying spare tubes, patch kits, tire levers, keys and some extra money. Some saddle bags are small, and others are larger. These can be found in bike stores or department stores. A saddle bag is a standard necessity for your bike.

WATER BOTTLE AND CAGES

If you are buying a bike from a local bike store, they may throw in a plastic water bottle and cage to sweeten the deal, if you're a person that likes to haggle. It does not hurt to ask!

Water bottles used to serve as the primary way for riders to hydrate, but now they are mostly for backup water. I say this because riders now use a hydration pack instead. If you are going to use frame mounted water bottles as your primary source of water, it is necessary, in my rationale, to buy sport bottles that have a finger release cap spout cover. If you really think about it, bicycle water bottles are located a few inches from both tires. Logically, that means any watery gutter spray your tires spit out (and they do) is spattered on the mouthpiece of your bottles. YUCK! I don't feel confident putting them to my mouth!

In addition to gutter spray, as you may have noticed, paved city trails have an abundance of green slimy spit balls that are scattered abroad from runners. And after the rain, this super gross mixture of runner phlegm and mucky rainwater goes on your tires and will most definitely end up on your bottles. Super Yuck! GERMS! So, buy your bottles with a mouthpiece cap! And BPA free too. Or, better yet, buy a hydration pack, and only use any bottles connected to your bike frame as backup in extreme cases or to wash hands (a full description of the hydration pack can be found in Chapter 5, **HYDRATION PACK**).

As for bottle cages, plastic ones are very inexpensive these days and can be found at department stores and even at dollar stores.

TIP 1 – It is a good idea to buy a mister. You may be able to find one that fits into a water bottle cage. On hot days, as the body starts to overheat, a mister is a great tool to cool down and refresh. As summer ends, these are reduced to clear, like all summer items. So, buy two and be prepared, since hot weather is still not over, and there is always next summer!

TIP 2 – A water bottle can double as a tool kit. Simply purchase a bottle (one that will not be used for drinking) that has a wide cap (and wide neck) and put all your tools in it. This works well and keeps all your tools in an easy-to-get-to place. A water bottle can also be used to store thin extra tubes. Don't reuse any water bottle used for storing tools or tubes for drinking.

BAR ENDS

Bar Ends seem to go in and out of fashion and favor as far as I can tell. But, for any bike (with flat or riser bars) that you plan to ride uphill on with intensity, or speedily down a long road, bar-ends will help you do just that. Bar Ends allow a person to posture his or herself to muscle up by shifting a rider's weight. This front weight redistribution weighs down and grounds the front tire giving a person more leverage and traction on the incline. And on straight-a-ways, bar ends allow the rider an aerodynamic body positioning and a powerful grip option that favors force on the down stroke. Plus, they look cool too!

Bar Ends, being that they offer a different riding hand positioning, help with any hand numbness on a long ride. And if mated with grips with palm platforms or "wings," they become a winning combination. Typically, bar ends are sold in longer and shorter styles for one's preference and hand size. There are also sets made of composite material. These are more expensive than aluminum sets. Given these options, there is no reason to put up with only one hand position.

Overall, bar ends offer better comfort and more power than handlebars alone, and should not be dismissed as an old trend.

TIP 1 – Bar ends can be wrapped with handlebar tape. You can also cut-to-size old grips to cover them, making them more comfortable.

TIP 2 – Sometimes bar ends can slip from position on the handlebar. This is especially true with the composite ones, since the fastening bolt on them should not be tightened too tight. Here is a solution so you don't strip the inner nut. Simply put a latex glove over the handlebar end. Then slide the bar end in position over the glove. Tighten bolt and trim the rest of the glove off with a blade. Problem fixed!

NOTE: Stock bars or light performance cross-country bars for bar ends? I feel it is best to use stock aluminum handlebars if you are going to install bar ends on your bike. Why? Because stock bars have thicker walls than light performance trail/cross-country bars. They feel more stable. Performance bars can be double or triple butted, making the walls at the ends thin. This can make them feel flimsy and like they are going to fail in some way when used with bar ends. To me, it seems unlikely that ultra-thin bars can handle the torque of riding with bar ends. Opinions differ on this topic. You can ask your local bike shop or the handlebar manufacturer if you are in doubt.

What does "butted" mean in reference to bars or tubes? It basically means "thinned down to reduce weight".

BELL

I would not call a bell an absolute necessity. But it is a useful tool when going downhill on a mountain bike, to give hikers the heads up that you are coming through. Also, city trails are filled with walking slowpokes who need to be reminded that the paved lane is called a "bike path" for a reason. I think any device that brings awareness that there is a bike rider coming through is good. So, I would not look down on a bike bell as something cliché, or for kids. It has a legit purpose for riding, and that goes for adults, too. But, please, don't buy a squeeze horn; those are for clowns.

TIP – In choosing a bell, smaller is always better. A bell needs to be out of the way of the shifters and brake levers. There is not a lot of space there for a bell. So, choose it carefully.

NOTE: In recent times, bike bells have taken on more varieties. In fact, many companies have taken bell design to new levels, offering very well-made modern bells whose look and sound are not as the typical bells of yesteryear. They have been reinvented to appease a hipper, more sophisticated crowd of riders who frown on the old typical style, and need something better, something more urban modern. A contemporary reboot!

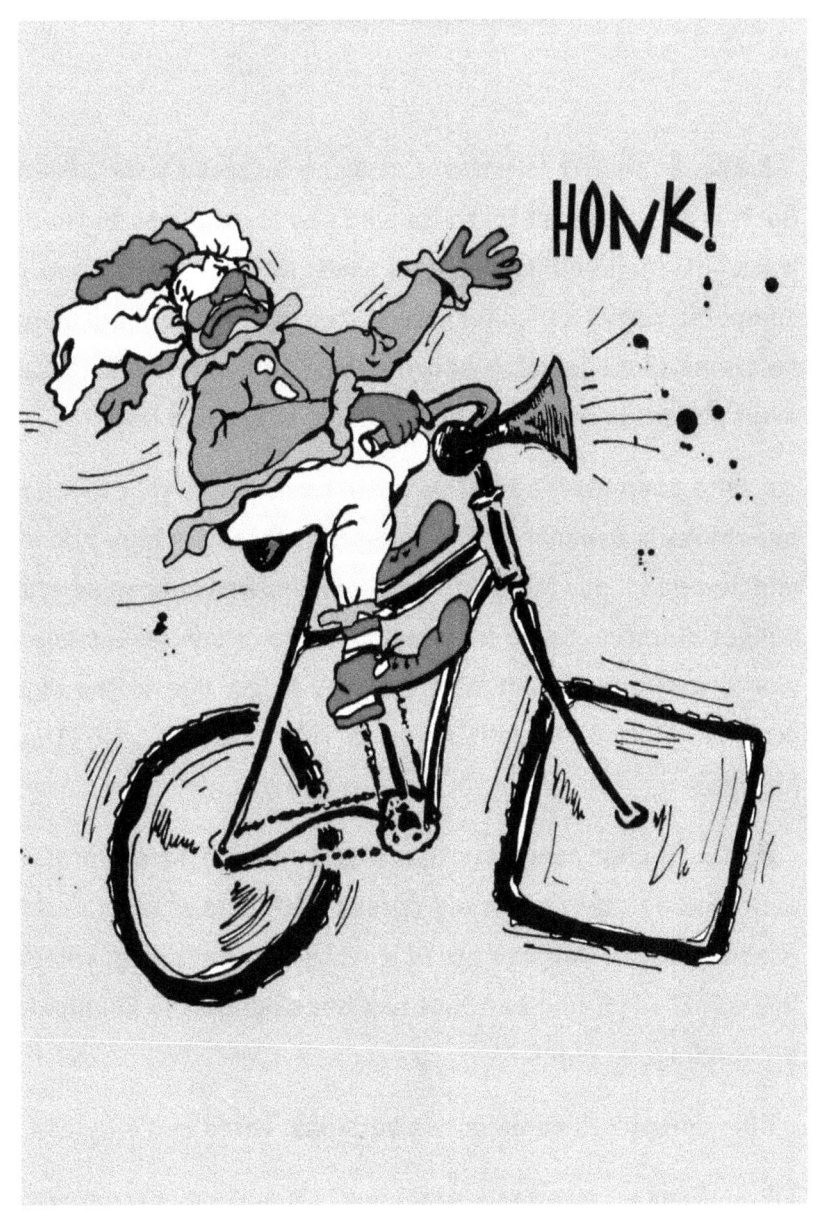

COMPUTER

A bike computer is not a necessary accessory for a bike. But it is a cool gadget for those who like to calculate and keep track of their riding exploits and riding information. A computer makes a bike look sharp and smart. There are many functions, like odometer, speedometer, present ride distance, average speed, ride time, and a clock, to name a few.

A bike computer is relative in its cost, contingent to what one thinks is expensive. But being that there are high-priced, middle-priced, and low-priced models, you can choose as your budget dictates. Some find buying a cheap one (assuming it works well and is accurate) the way to go, due to the high probability it might fall off on a ride and get lost. That happens!

Buying a bike computer that has a familiar name on it is safe, and one that has a big screen with bold readable print is necessary. If you can't read it while you are riding, what's the point? Also, find one that has back-lighting to illuminate the readings at night.

Bike computers come in two versions: wired and wireless.

TIP – Sensor accuracy problems? Mount your computer sensor and magnet 4 or 5 inches outward from the center of the wheel hub or just beyond where the spokes cross for better accuracy. The outer end of the wheel travels faster and this speed may mess with the gauging. Putting the magnet closer to the hub may help the sensor read it better. But as always, follow the instructions.

MIRROR

If you are going to do a lot of congested city riding, you should buy a bike mirror. A bike mirror will allow you to see behind the left of you without turning your head to look over your shoulder. There are many types of bike mirrors and many ways that they are attached.

Some strap on the handlebar grips and are removable. Others clamp on the bars close to the brakes and shifters. Still others clip to your glasses. And some are fastened to helmets. I use one that clips to my glasses. It works great! Here's the criterion for a good helmet or glasses-mounted mirror:

1) Large (relative), to reduce squinting.
2) Wide is better than round or square, for more road visibility.
3) Strong extension post, to reduce vibrations.
4) Good adjustability, for repositioning.

NOTE: I find the best position for a helmet mirror is further to the left and out of frontal vision. Also, further forward to reduce squinting and focusing issues. Improvise if necessary.

TIRE LINERS

These days, even on expensive bikes, I've noticed that the thickness of tires has been shaved down to as thin as they can get. Inner tubes seem to have followed suit. This makes for lightweight wheels, but it steals from a tire's ability to resist punctures. The solution to this problem are tire liners. Tire liners are not expensive. They offer tires additional protection from glass and thorns. They are not hard to install, fitting between the inner tire and tube. Tire liners come in different sizes and widths for your specific tire size. The only two downsides that I can think of are these:

1) Tire liners can take out the springy feel of a tire, making it feel kind of dull and lifeless. Most novice riders will not notice this, as they are not attuned to the minute nuances of their bike. But long-time riders will notice. This is worthy to note, but not a deal breaker.
2) Tire liners in a tire do have some extra overlap where one end meets the other. This flap of overlap, after much riding, rubs against and wears into the tube. And over time, it will cause a flat. I have experienced this firsthand. But if you are a handy person, you can fix this altogether. Simply round (if not already) and bevel (taper) the end of the liner that overlaps and comes in contact with the tube. Round it with scissors. After, sand the

edges smooth. Then, with a file or sandpaper bevel or thin down the end of the liner so it will not protrude and press into the tube. This should take care of the problem! Remember that tire liners are not guaranteed flat protection. They are only extra protection.

TIP – Clean off your tire liner after fixing a flat. Sometimes there are bits of inner tire shavings and tiny rocks sticking to them. These can rub the surface of a tube and create a hole. Also, make sure there are no thorns embedded in the tire, inside and out, or any stuck in the liner itself.

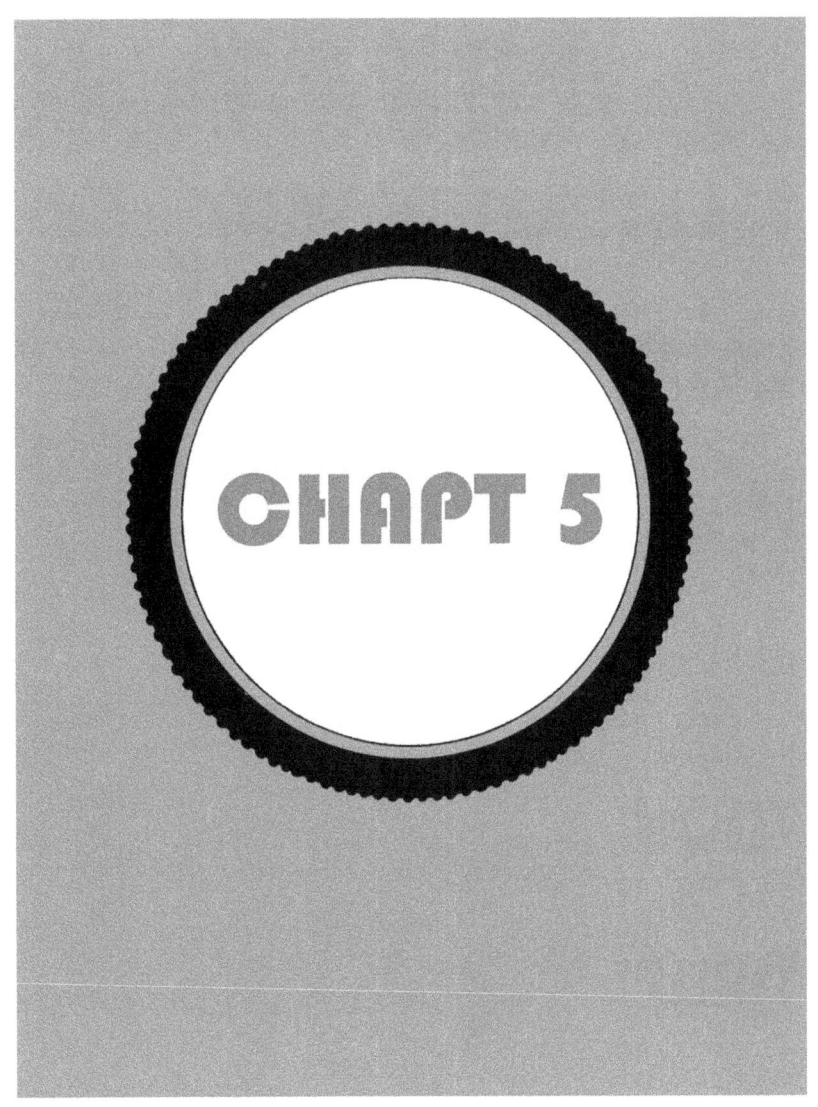

PACK SMART - THE ART OF WHAT TO BRING

THE HYDRATION PACK

WATER

FOOD

MEDICAL KIT

TOOLS

TUBES

PATCH KIT

MONEY

MISCELLANEOUS

HYDRATION PACK

In this chapter, I am going to address the main things that a rider is going to have to bring along with him/her in order to be reasonably equipped for whatever comes his/her way. This is an art, because there are many things that a person thinks of bringing along, but the chances that you are really going to need them are remote. So, it takes a bit of experience to understand what you <u>will</u> need, what you <u>might</u> need and what you really <u>don't</u> need. A rider always needs to keep weight to a minimum.

Today's riders carry most of what they need in their hydration pack. This is a light narrow backpack, designed for the rider's needs, that has a built-in water unit consisting of a bladder (to hold the water), tube, and mouthpiece for drinking water or sports drinks. It usually has some storage compartments (more on this later) to carry other items that cyclists must bring along, in addition to just water.

Your hydration pack is not a bug out bag. It is not meant to survive the zombie apocalypse. It is for a selective set of minimal items specifically chosen for riding purposes. It must be well thought out and light. So, in this section I will discuss the things in my experience that a rider is going to have to bring along. This list is general, but adequate for over-all riding, and can be personally tailored to each rider's individual needs. But first, let's talk packs.

CHOOSING THE RIGHT PACK

In a world of choices, there is a plethora of hydration pack brands and manufacturers to choose from. There are big bicycle gear brands, sport gear brands, and no-name makers out there. Big bicycle gear brands (found in bike stores) design their packs with the cyclist and his/her special needs in mind (pricey). Sport gear brands and no-name brands and makers (found in department stores) cater to a more nonspecific and general sport enthusiast (relatively inexpensive). But they all share the same commonality of materials they are made from and general features. So, in that, they are all on equal footing, setting aside any objections one might have over design particulars and opinions on durability. Remember, no pack lasts forever, not even the most expensive, and the life expectancy to a pack can be anywhere from 3 to 5 years (depending on use). So, don't obsess too much about it; you'll be replacing it relatively quick.

To me, the bigger issue is not the brand or price, but a basic feature that is cyclist specific. This feature is namely the secondary storage compartment. A pack that can only accommodate a water bladder is useless to a bike rider, because a cyclist obviously needs a second compartment to carry other things. And this compartment needs to be of about

EQUAL size to that which holds the water. This should be number one in a cyclist hydration pack. Not all hydration packs are created equal in this department. Also, a chest strap and waist strap are necessary features.

A hydration pack should not have tricky vertical side zipping pockets and small compartments on it. Vertical side zipping pockets can unzip, and as a result you'll lose stuff on a ride. And small compartments and the likes only confuse the bag. So, purchase one with horizontal zippers to the top and a simple design.

NOTE 1: I do not recommend using a hip pack in place of a hydration pack if you are a male, although many riders use them. The reasons being these:

1) Males have narrow hips and not much butt to hold the pack up to the waist, consequently the pack just keeps sliding down no matter how tight you make the strap (which makes it highly uncomfortable). In addition, most riders wear spandex shorts, which are smooth. This only increases the slipping. So, a weighty mid-sized pack will be an utter nuisance to keep in place, and will just hang down the duration of the ride. "Been there, done that!" These hip packs are better suited for females due to their wider hips and smaller waist, which keeps the pack in place.

2) Hip packs are relatively small in relation to a shoulder held backpack, although they vary in size. Most can't even hold half the contents of an average hydration pack.

And if you do find a large one, then you're back to reason 1, slipping. So, ditch these. They are only useful to a male in carrying a wallet, keys and some nutrition bars.

NOTE 2: They do make a hip pack that has shoulder straps in addition to a waist strap. This might work well. But to me, it does not solve the problem of its size compared to a hydration pack.

NOTE 3: On a negative note, the shoulder and chest straps on a hydration pack can cause scuff patterns around the area of the cycling jersey they rest upon. This is due to the constant swinging movement of the pack that occurs while riding. Not all hydration packs do this, but some do. So, wear your best jersey when you are not using a hydration pack.

NOTE 4: A rider should not carry any items in the bladder compartment if the bladder is inside, filled or unfilled. Items packed on or near the bladder can puncture the bladder.

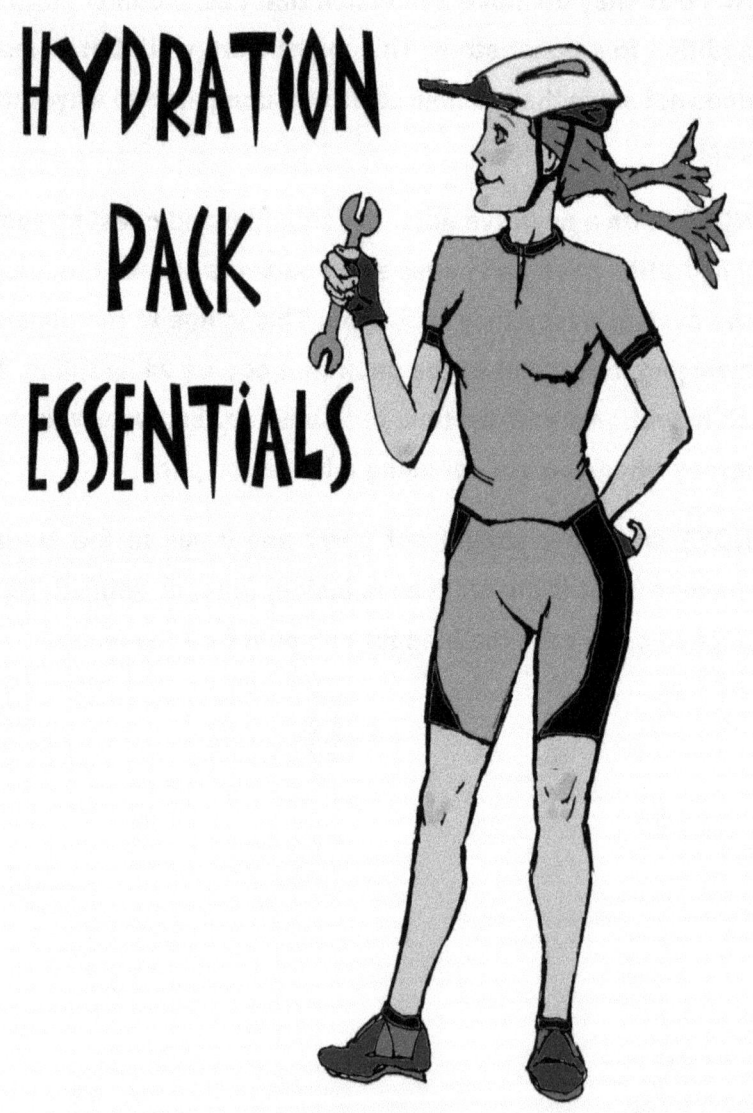

PACK ESSENTIALS

Keep in mind that one should be organized and know exactly where to find what they need, when they need it. It is a bad idea to pour out the contents of your pack on the ground and shuffle around looking for something in particular. So, it is especially important to keep the items in your hydration pack in separate organized color-coded pouches and specifically marked. This will ensure things are faster to find, and are clean, and safe if there is a leak. You can also use zip-lock freezer bags bought at a dollar store. They come in many sizes.

Nylon zippered pouches will do well for the job. These can be bought at department stores where they carry school supplies. A variety of these will be found in late July thru September before school begins. Write with a marker on each pouch the category of its contents, such as:

1) Tools
2) Food
3) Medical kit
4) Money (If you do not have a wallet inside)

Here are some things you will need to pack in an easy-to-get-to place in your hydration pack. Some are mentioned further on as part of a bigger list, but these items ought to be put where you can get to them relatively quickly and with no hassle.

1) A small pencil (or pen) and some paper. You might need to jot down some information or a phone number. Brilliant ideas sometimes flash into your mind and need to be remembered, as epiphanies do come while you are on a ride.
2) Two packets of tissues. These can be used for cleaning cuts, runny noses, restroom stops and to clean hands.
3) A small bottle of hand sanitizer. Hand sanitizer is needed if you accidentally come in contact with something gross.
4) Disposable Gloves. These can be worn to treat a wound or to keep your hands clean if you have a chain malfunction or a dirty flat. Pack at least two pairs in a resealable plastic bag. Replace any latex, nitrile, or vinyl gloves regularly, because they break down over time. Nitrile gloves will store longer than latex and vinyl.
5) Tuck a small tube of sunscreen in your pack. Better safe than burnt.
6) Light disposable rain poncho (if in rainy season).
7) Wallet with money and identification.
8) Pepper spray (protection).
9) Pocketknife.

Remember to always think compact and light!
Now, let's go further into the essentials of a well-prepared hydration pack.

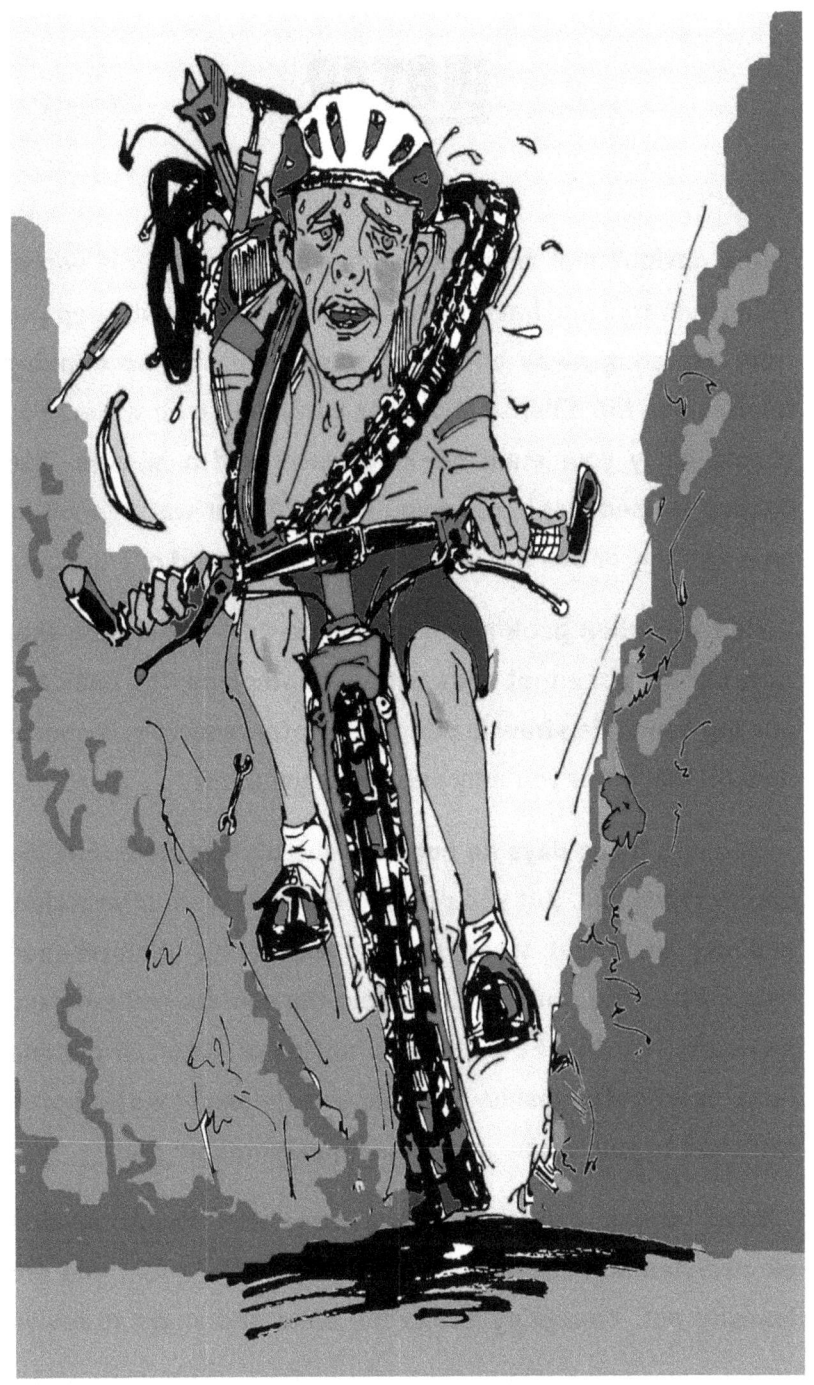

WATER

One obvious and most basic thing a rider needs is water. Being hydrated and having a source of hydration will keep you from withering away on a long ride. There are no drinking fountains in the hills, so you must carry your own water. You should carry your main drinking water and a backup. The backup is used just in case you drink all your water, such as on a hot day, or can be used to clean an injury if one occurs.

Your hydration pack has a bladder inside, and a tube that runs out the pack that ends with a mouthpiece. It's basically one big bendable straw leading to a water reservoir. It should hold all the water you may need on a good ride.

Bladders these days do not have the plastic taste that the earlier types had. But you do have to clean them after a ride, and dry them out when not in use. If the maintenance becomes a drag, you could take out the bladder and tube and just carry two 16.9 FL OZ plastic bottles of water. Or put one large sport bottle inside. You can use the usual water bottle attached to your frame as the backup. Works for me!

Sport drinks are good. They can offer much needed electrolytes and sugar, saving the day in the event you are bonking out. Your body needs the salts and sugar to revive and replenish quickly. There are many brands of sport drinks. They all serve the same purpose, hydration!

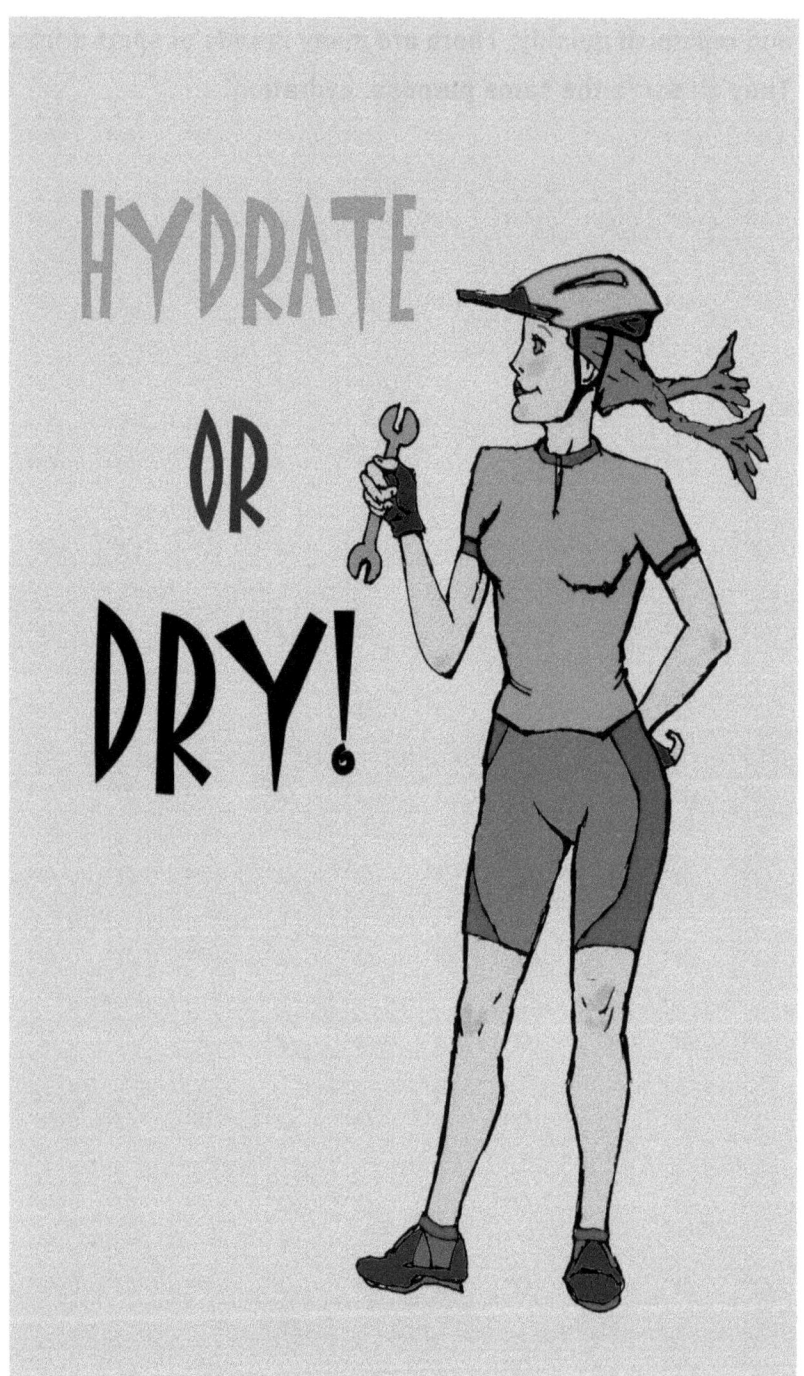

FOOD

You have been riding for a while and are beginning to bonk out. Your legs feel like rubber and your head, dizzy and jittery. You need some calories, and quick, but all you brought was water. This is a novice mistake, right? I guess you could knock on someone's door, if you are near a house, and ask for a candy bar as a last resort. This obviously would be a ridiculous, desperate act. Better to simply bring some nutrition bars with you. Carrying nutrition bars is especially necessary if you are a mountain biker riding the hills. Last time I checked there was no convenient store nestled in the rocks. Normally, you will eat and feel energized before you start a ride, but those calories will eventually get used up.

I rode up a long winding canyon road one day, feeling energized. After the climb to the top, I bonked out. I did not bring any food or nutrition bars with me. It was a spur of the moment ride. Dizzy and shaky, I considered all my options. After searching what I had on me, I found a small pack of old raisins I had forgotten in my saddle bag. Eating those stale raisins gave me just enough energy to get home. The only other options were to knock on a stranger's door or to eat a squirrel. What would you do?

Back in the day, riders carried a banana or two in a large pocket situated in the back of their cycle jersey. That's why jerseys are still made with pockets. Although, it is conceivable and highly likely early riders probably used them for spare tubes or extra water bottles as well. It seems ridiculous to us now that all they had were bananas! Then came "gorp," a combination of loose granola, chocolate bits, peanuts, raisins and whatever, in a plastic bag. That worked somewhat, if the chocolate didn't create a gooey mess wherever you hid it. But it lacked sufficient protein. Then there were granola-based bars, which were convenient, but lacked protein too. These were snack bars and marketed as such. And now, there are nutrition bars! There is a grand assortment of well-balanced, individually packed bars that address nutrition.

Most of these bars are designed to give a balance of calories, protein, and salt, to get you back into the race. Many are "gluten free" or whatever "free" you need. So, there is absolutely no reason not to have a few in your pack. Buy some! Put your bars (about three of them) in the food pouch in your pack to keep the wrappers from getting punctured. Also, replace them regularly to keep them fresh. Small packs of assorted nuts, seeds and raisins are also good.

One time I had some granola bars in a backpack in my truck. I felt that I needed some energy and opened one, finding it was covered with worms. All the others I had were infested with worms, too. So, unless you like to eat worms, its best to switch them out often.

TIP 1 – Try to avoid bars that have chocolate. They will melt and make a big gooey mess inside of your pack if punctured.

TIP 2 – It is probably not a good idea to use beef jerky in your hydration pack as food. High protein requires a lot of water to digest. And this eaten before or during a ride will make you thirsty and use up your water for the ride.

TIP 3 – Bring along a plastic camping combination fork/spoon (keep it in a sealable plastic bag). This is for urgent market stops. Yogurt or canned fruit can be bought as a cheap and quick pick-me-up food. And there's never a spoon around when you need one. So, pack your own.

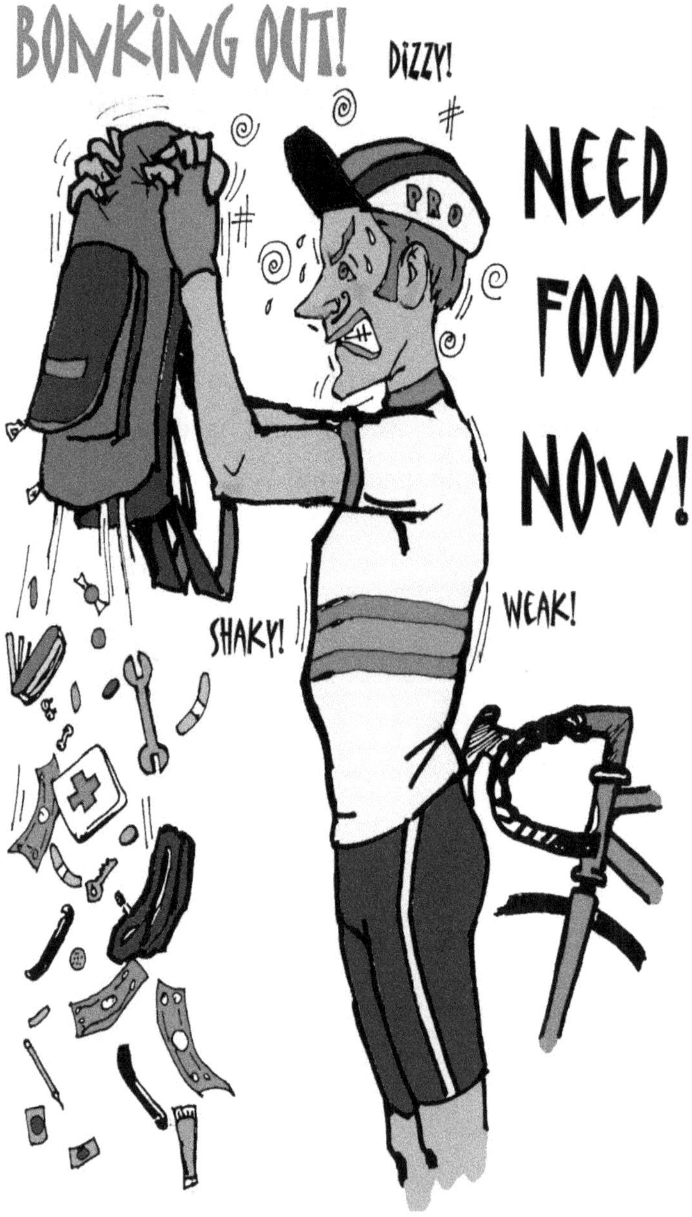
BONKING OUT!
DIZZY!
NEED FOOD NOW!
PRO
SHAKY!
WEAK!

MEDICAL KIT

A medical kit is one of the most necessary items to have and should not be skimped on. Most of the things that are contained in it are light and flat. So, you can stuff it with all the things you need and not have to be concerned with weight and space.

Your medical kit should be well stocked for big scrapes, minor cuts, and even deep punctures. Most injuries come from falling off a bike or from a hit to the shin by the pedals. All bike injuries will need a good amount of cleaning, especially if they have had contact with the dirty street or dusty trail. A hit from the pedal to the shin can be quite deep and bloody. So, be prepared.

Another common trail injury is caused by spikes of various kinds. There are cactus thorns, weed thorns, wood splinters, and weed prickles. If one or many get lodged in your skin, you'll need some tweezers, a small magnifying glass, and a clean needle (optional) to remove it/them. So, these items will be considered basics in your medical kit. Keep them in a clean place in your kit. Store any needle taped inside a small plastic container where there is no chance of it poking through your pack.

Here is a list of basic things you should put in your medical kit:

1) Large and small band aids.

2) Antiseptic spray and gel. You need both for different applications.

3) Disposable gloves (two pair), to keep any cut clean and free from touching with dirty hands. Also, you may need to treat a scrape on someone else.

4) Tweezers, small magnifying glass, and a needle (optional).

5) Aspirin (serving size packets).

6) 2 Packs of tissues.

7) Medical tape or self-adhesive elastic wrap (to hold any large bandage in place).

8) Disposable lighter (to sterilize tweezers and needle).

9) 3 small Wing bandages (for a gaping wound).

10) 3 Cough drops (optional).

11) Disinfectant wipes.

12) Liquid bandage.

13) Small mirror.

14) Lip balm.

15) Breath mints (optional).

16) Whistle.

17) Small packs of wet wipes.

18) Extra pair of prescription glasses (If you use some).

19) Small liquid soap bottle (for long day trips).

TIP 1 – If you are on any medications, it is a good idea to include it or them too. Be sure to keep it or them in the original prescription bottle.

TIP 2 – As I mentioned, most cycling scrapes and cuts occur at or below the knee, most commonly by falling off your bike or taking a hit to the shin. In addition to the initial injury, which can get infected, there is a secondary risk of infection due to road debris and germ loaded gutter water splashing on a cut as you get back on the road. Roads are dirty, and that should be clear to every rider. So, clean and disinfect any wound that has occurred and **COVER WELL** before riding again. Do not leave any part of the wound uncovered. Also, avoid any puddles or wet roads along the way. And when you get home, repeat the cleaning and disinfecting and don't ride again till the open wound heals.

TOOLS

MULTI-TOOLS: THE SKINNY

Tools are an interesting thing to contemplate, and are one of the necessary tackle in your hydration pack. Since they are made of metal, and metal is heavy, the tools you take with you must be well thought out in both weight and practicality. Here I will endeavor to break it down in understandable and reasonable thinking.

Back in the day, cyclists carried their tools loosely jangling in their saddle bag or in a roll out pocketed nylon thingy. But now we have multi-tools. A multi-tool is a folding assortment of tools that is compact and capable of meeting all cyclist repair needs on the road. These small multi-tools are the standard in cycling road tools. They also should not be considered optional. But wait! Don't run to the hardware or sporting goods store just yet and buy any old multi-tool, thinking it will do the job. These general multi-tools would not be equipped with anything that would be helpful in fixing a bike. The type you need must be **DESIGNED SPECIFICALLY** for bike repair. So, making sure your tool is made for cycling is foremost. And beyond that, there are even more particulars.

You basically want your multi-tool to be equipped with tools that you need and not be filled superfluously with nonsense gismos for the sake of looking "cool." You don't need cork screws, bottle openers, nail files or a saw blade. You want it to have only what you need to fix your bike. And you want it light and small!

It is also particularly important to make sure that your multi-tool contains tools that are applicable to your specific bike. Some multi-tools (mainly department store ones) may have a range of tools that are for older and more basic bikes, such as tools to tighten older hexagon bolt heads. The bolts on standard newer bikes require Allen wrenches to tighten them. So, it is a waste of space and weight to carry anything other than Allen wrenches for bolts. Scrutinize every item on a multi-tool. Multi-tools vary greatly in both the combinations of implements and quantity. Your multi-tool must be minimal, applicable, and light.

Here's a quick list of essential necessities for your multi-tool:

1) Both types of screwdrivers.
2) Allen wrenches for every bolt on your bike, including crank bolts.
3) Chain breaker tool.
4) Spoke tool (one that fits your spokes).

NOTE: Some multi-tools come with a large assortment of spoke tool sizes. This is an unnecessary waste of space and added weight, considering you need only one size. It's far better to have a multi-tool that does not have any spoke tools in it, and just carry a separate spoke tool (your size).

Further, if your bike has bolt-on wheels, it would be necessary to find a multi-tool having a light, adjustable crescent wrench in it. Good luck on that! They used to make at least one multi-tool for cyclists that had a crescent wrench, but I haven't seen any version of one for a while.

Here are some other things that are a good idea to carry in your tool pouch:

1) Medium zip-ties.
2) Separate micro-tool with pliers (to safely pull nails and thorns out of tires).
3) Small length of chain (for spare parts in the event of a chain break).
4) Small pocketknife.
5) Chain hook (holds chain together for repairs).

NOTE: Your hydration pack tools should not be your primary tools that you use on your bike. These are for fixing things on the road. As mentioned in Chapter 2, under **YOUR TOOLBOX**, you should have a large toolbox for your bike. This should be kept separate from your house tools.

Main Tools recap:

1) Bicycle multi-tool (bike tools only).
2) Micro-tool (with pliers).
3) Small pocketknife.

TUBES

Ideally, you should carry two tubes with you. You may think that is overkill, but it's not. One day I rode to a church that was near a hill. After service I decided to ride my mountain bike up the hill and enjoy the view. While riding the dirt trail beside the street, I heard crunching sounds. Looking down at my tires, to my surprise I saw that they were completely covered in goathead weed thorns. I also heard hissing sounds.

After walking my bike to a place where I could assess the problem, I began to pull thorns. I pulled out about 300 thorns between my front tire and back. Yes, I counted them. Even with tire liners, the number of holes in my tubes was unbelievable. I had one tube and some patches with me. I did not happen to carry 300 patches with me that day ... ha, ha. So, I put in the spare tube and did the best I could patching up the other tube.

To make a long story short, to get home, I had to stop just about every block and inflate my tire. That was a pain! So, the moral of the story is, BRING TWO TUBES! If you bring two tubes, you are guaranteed to be able to fix a flat of even 300 thorns and ride home. You only need two. You can divide two tubes between your saddle bag and your hydration pack if your saddle bag can't hold two. Spare tubes can also be attached to the frame of your bike.

And one important piece of advice: if you are storing a tube in your saddle bag, keep your tube in its original plastic, or if it has none, put it in a sock. Why? Because as you ride, the constant bobbing up and down, and side to side, will rub the pointed folded ends of the tube against the inside of the bag, eventually putting holes in the tube. So, you'll take out your tube only to find it needing patches as well. Been there, done that, too!

SCHRADER VS. PRESTA VALVES

Tubes have valves. These valves are used to inflate or deflate the tube, and come in two types. The standard type is called a Schrader valve, like the type on cars and motorcycle tires. The other type is the Presta valve (The French Valve), which is thinner and has a much different valve design than that of the Schrader.

Your choice of tube valve type is somewhat decided by your rims. Rims are made to have a certain type of valve. A rim made for a Schrader valve will have a large rim hole that can also accommodate the Presta type, because the width of a Presta valve is smaller. The Presta will fit a bit loosely in it, but there are inserts available that will hold the valve snug. A rim made for a Presta valve, on the other hand, will have a smaller valve hole. So, if you want to run a Schrader valve type tube, you will have to drill out the hole with a 21/64 drill bit, making it bigger. Visit your bike shop to make sure your rim is strong enough to drill.

I have warmed up to the Presta valve over the Schrader in recent years. I like the mechanics of it. The Schrader to me is outdated, bulky, and you always need some sort of pointed object to press down the inner needle to deflate it. Not so with the Presta valve. It has a screw-down nut mechanism that can handle high pressure. It is sporty, sleeker, and easy to deflate by itself. My vote is for the Presta!

HOW TO CHANGE A TUBE

You are having a good time riding your bike on a bright sunny day, just minding your own business. Then you hear that dreaded sound, SSSSSSSS, and cry out, Nooooo!!!! Why me?!!! Your tire is becoming flat. What do you do?

Pull off to a place that is out of the sunlight, and if possible, has some grass. If you have disposable gloves, put them on. It can be messy if it is the back tire, due to the chain.

First thing is to remove the wheel. But before you do, do this. If it is the back tire that has the flat, make sure you switch your gears to the smallest cog in the rear and the largest chainring in the front. This is very important. Many new riders don't know that this needs to be done. If you don't do this first, you will spend much time in frustration trying to slide out the rear wheel, and won't be able to. Why? Because your rear derailleur and chain will be in the way; their position will not let you remove the wheel until they are shifted more out of the way. This applies to reinstalling the wheel as well. Now, the steps to fix a flat:

1) If your bike has a V-brake system, you must release the noodle out of the noodle holder. This will disengage the brake arms so the brakes can open and the tire can be pulled through the pads. After that is done, turn the wheel quick-release lever outward and unscrew it just enough to remove the wheel. Remove your wheel with the skewer rod still in the hub and halfway bolted (if you unscrew the skewer fully, you may lose the springs).

2) Now that the wheel is removed, push one tire lever between the tire and the rim and begin to unseat the tire bead (lip) in that spot. Once the bead is over the rim, lock the lever into place with the hook-like projection located at the lever's other end. Attach it (straight wise) to the nearest outward-facing spoke, and make sure it is secure, so it won't fling out.

3) Insert the other lever the same way about a few inches away, and begin to unseat the bead there too. Once the tire bead is over the rim in that spot, slide that lever along the whole rim. Unseat the entire tire bead on that side disconnecting the first lever as you meet it. Try not to pinch or tear the tube. If the tire side is difficult to unseat, you can use a third lever to assist.

4) Now, after fully unseating one side of the tire from the wheel, pull out the tube. Examine the outside of the tire for the source of the flat. Then, visually inspect the inside. **IDENTIFY THE SOURCE OF THE PUNCTURE BEFORE TOUCHING THE INSIDE OF THE TIRE.** Do this slowly. (See also Chapter 7, under **STRANGE ROAD**

HAZARDS.) You will probably find the thorn that penetrated the tire. There may be more than one. Pull out the thorn from the outside of the tire. Pull it with the micro-tool's pliers. Make sure you pull out all of it.

5) Now, put some air in the tube and listen for the **SSSSSSSS**.
6) Apply a patch (the patch application procedure is detailed in the next section).
7) After you patch the hole, inflate the tube just enough that it has some form, and place it back in the tire. Now seat the side of the tire back into the rim. This can be done with your fingers if you have fat tires. If not, use the tire levers to lift the bead (lip) over the rim and back in, and be careful not to pinch the tube.
8) After the tire is fully on, inflate to where it barely takes shape and is soft. Now squeeze the sides (full circumference, both sides) of the tire and inspect the bead. Make sure the tube is out of the way of the tire bead and rim. If any part of the tube is caught between the tire bead and rim it will very likely blow upon inflation. Massage the sides of the tire (full circumference) to help the entire tire seat better. Next, you're good to go on inflating. After inflating to desired **PSI**, reinstall the wheel on the bike and tighten the wheel quick-release lever just enough to where the wheel won't fall out. Reattach the brake noodle back in the noodle holder. Now, center the wheel. Once the wheel is centered (between the brake pads), you can tighten the

lever all the way. Remember, when tightening a quick release, resistance should start between fully open and fully locked for proper tension.

BEWARE OF THE EVIL WEED!

Goathead weed (AKA, Puncturevine or Tribulus Terrestris) is the biggest menace to any mountain biker's tires, second to none. It is the tire tube killer! This flat greenish mat-like weed with yellow flowers grows in loose soil and does not stand out from its surroundings. Its flower (seedhead) contains a cluster of barbed thorns that can pierce through a tire down to the tube without any problem. As the weed dries (late in the year), the thorns harden (and break off) and the weed becomes a treacherous bed containing **HUNDREDS** of these very sharp thorny monsters. The bush is practically invisible, that is, until you ride over it. Then it's too late!

Removing these nasty thorns out of a tire requires strong tweezers (or small pliers), patience, and thick skin. You, no doubt, will prick yourself in the process (a lot!).

It is advisable to become familiar with this weed and keep your eyes peeled for it. Understand that evasion is your only defense against it. For it is truly the weed from **HELL!**

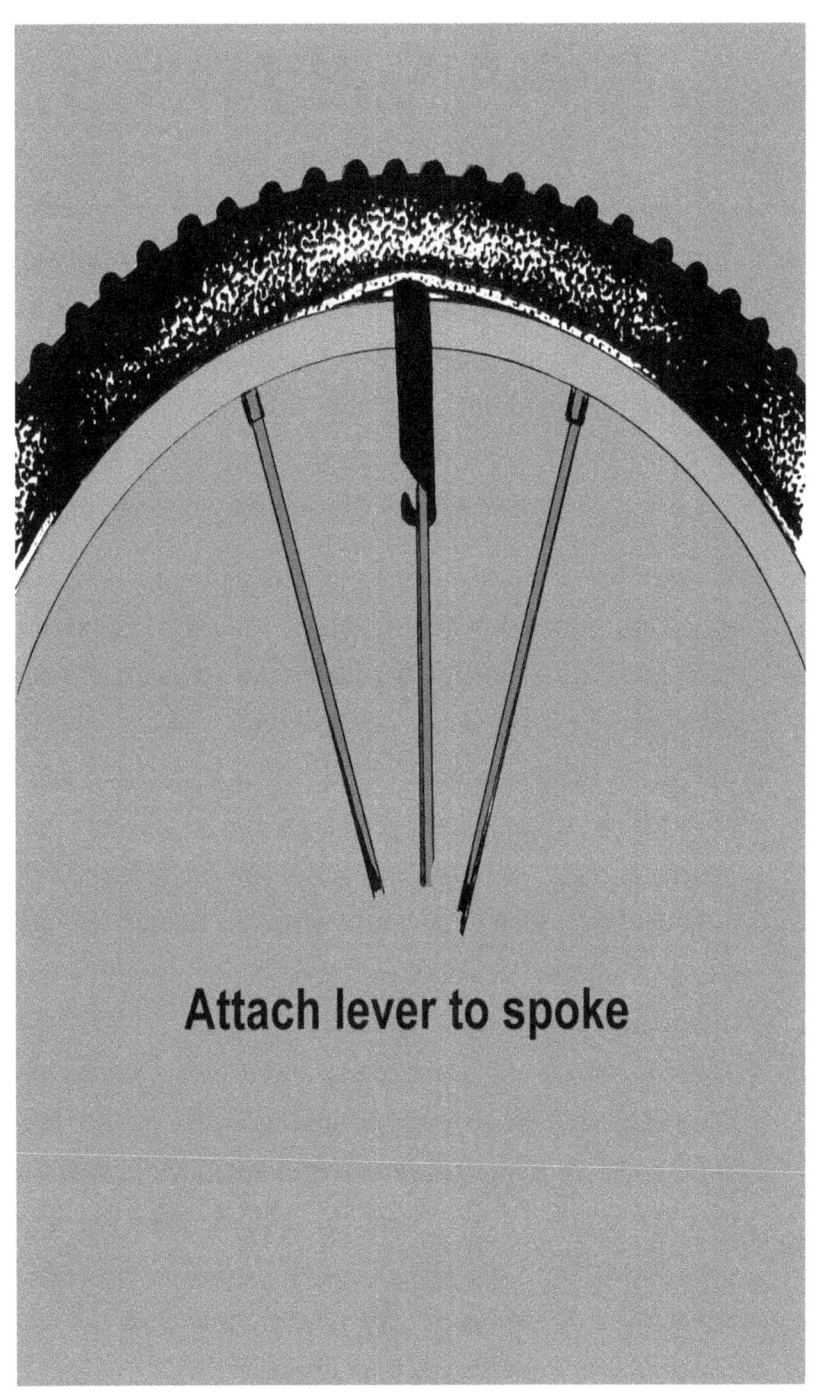
Attach lever to spoke

MY TIRE WON'T SEAT RIGHT!

After you fix a flat and fill up the tire, spin it and check if there are any low points in the tire as it spins. A tire must be seated properly in the rim. If the tire is seating more deeply in one spot of the rim, the result will be a flat spot in that area. Its tread will go up and down when the wheel is spun. And if you ride it in this condition, your bike, with you on it, will bob up and down too, making for a miserable ride. So, if you do notice a low point in one side of the tire, do these things:

1) Remove tire and check if the rim strip (a plastic or rubber strip that runs along the center of the rim) is centered correctly. If it even slightly runs up the side of the inside of the rim, your tire will not seat right.

2) Deflate the tire to almost empty and massage the sides of the tire at the bead. Massage the whole tire and manually pull it outward from the rim as you go. This releases any of the tire from sticking to the rim and allows the bead to equally align to the circle of the rim. Inflate and check the progress.

3) You can also brush some soapy water (not a lot) on the bead of the tire where the low spot is, below the rim line. Then pump to a higher-than-normal amount of air in the tire. There may be a popping sound when the tire seats. Then lower the pressure to normal. Do this in an open unenclosed area due to the slight chance of the tire blowing. Don't overdo the high pressure!

4) Your tube, for whatever reason, may not be filling up uniformly. That can be fixed by removing the tube and putting some air in it and gently and **SLIGHTLY** pulling on the opposite sides of the narrowing area at the same time. The narrowing area in the middle will expand.
5) The bike shop has a tool to pull the low spot out.
6) Sometimes a patched area will not expand (upon inflation) uniformly. The patch will not let the area inflate fully and it will taper causing a low spot. The only fix is to try a new tube.

PATCH KIT

There are two kinds of patches, the glue type and the glueless type. The glue type is typically the standard, as far as permanent repairs are concerned. It consists of glue, patches, and a scraping tool. The non-glue type, on the other hand, offers a quick, no-mess choice for fixing a flat. It includes only peel off patches and a scraping tool.

In recent years, I have found the glueless patches to be just as good and permanent as the glue type. I carry these with me on my rides. The glue in the tube of the glue types can evaporate and dry, leaving you in a sorry state if you have a flat. So, the glueless patches are definitely more reliable.

Tire levers must be a part of your patch kit. The plastic types are best because they are light and have little chance of scratching your rim. They also have less of a chance of damaging your tube if they pinch it. It is wise to carry three levers with you if you know your tires are normally hard to remove. This is usually the case on thin, high-pressure tires. Levers are not expensive, and cheap levers often break. So, buy good ones.

TIP 1 – When fixing a flat, make sure to secure the lever to the spoke, with its hook at the end of it, firmly and not haphazardly. A lever can fling and be a projectile if it is not secured right. Protect your eyes.

TIP 2 – If you have no patches and have a flat, you can cut the tube in two at the point of the puncture and tie each end in a knot. After putting the tube in the tire, inflate it. It may hold air long enough to get you home. If the puncture is near the tube valve, however, this is not an option. You can also fill your tire with grass. Or, best of all, call a friend to pick you up!

TIP 3 – A flat can be caused by a broken rim strip. The spoke nipple can poke into the tube from the inside. Be sure to inspect your rim strip as you fix your flat.

PATCH APPLICATION PROCEDURE

There is not much to putting on a patch. Fill the tube with some air and listen. Run your hand along the tube and feel for escaping air. Find it, and with a pen (always carry a pen in your pack) draw a 1-inch circle around the puncture (puncture being in the center). Let the air out and rough up the area in the circle with the scraper. After, make sure you brush off any tube scrapings and dust. Apply a thin layer of glue over the rough spot, not too much. Let the glue dry for two minutes till it looks dull. Then, peel off the back foil protective layer on the patch, trying not to touch the sticky part. Apply the patch over the scraped circle, hole in center, and press on it for a minute. Peel off the clear front plastic. Now you're good to go, as far as patching is concerned. In the case of the glueless type, forgo putting glue on the rough spot. Just peel the backing off the patch, stick the patch on the rough spot, and press well. Done!

TIP 1 – If you are at home, you can put a tube under water to find any punctures or leaks. Sometimes a leak will be found coming from a patch that is ungluing. Designate a bucket for this cause.

TIP 2 – It is good to keep used, patched up tire tubes as backups, and use them as chainstay protectors, as mentioned earlier.

TIP 3 – If for some reason, while on a ride, a chunk of tire tread falls off or rips, creating a small hole, you have a big problem. Stop immediately! Otherwise, some of the tire tube will bulge out of the hole, if it hasn't already. It will look like an odd black marble stuck to your tire. If you ride on it, the tube will immediately rupture and pop! Obviously, it is ridiculous to carry a spare tire. But there is a cheap and simple solution.

Find a soft plastic milk bottle. Then cut some rectangular and square (rounded edges) patches, about 1x2-inch for road and hybrid bikes and about 2x2-inch for mountain bikes. In the event this happens, simply put one of these plastic liners inside the tire between the inner tire and tube, where the hole is. This will prevent the tube from protruding out of the tire and protect it so you can ride home. So, make some and keep them handy in your patch kit. Also, make a patch with a slight curving bend to it, in case the tire mishap is to the side of the tire.

TIP 4 – Do not use a screwdriver or a knife as a tire lever. Any sharp object will likely puncture, pinch, or tear the tube.

TIP 5 – Old tire tubes can also be used as chain covers for a chain lock. Simply cut a tube two inches smaller than the size of the chain, wash out the powder inside, and let dry. Slip the chain through the tube. Done!

NOTE 1: I purchased a bike-store bike and got a flat on the first ride. I made several attempts at patching it, even using both types of patches. The patches would not adhere to the tube. I called the bike store to inquire as to why the patches would not stick. The shop person did not know. My guess is that tube manufacturers are experimenting with a different formula or materials to make their tubes. I ended up buying a new tube. Keep this in mind, it can happen!

NOTE 2: As mentioned earlier, if you store your bike indoors, lower the pressure of both tires before you go inside. Also, inflate your tires outdoors, and not indoors, or in any enclosed area. A tire blowout can cause injury in an enclosed area.

NOTE 3: If you run out of patch glue and patches, you can use rubber cement and patches made of an old tube. Simply cut a patch size square out of an old tube. Then, wash off any inner tube powder on the square. Scuff the side of the patch that will rest over the hole. Then scuff the area around the hole of the flat tube. Apply like any glue patch.

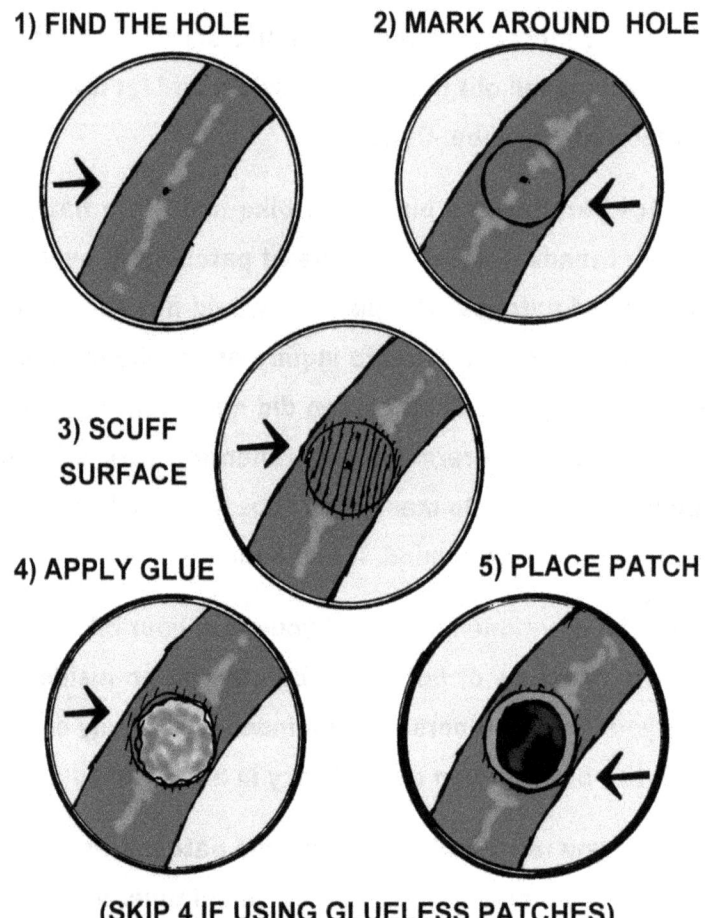

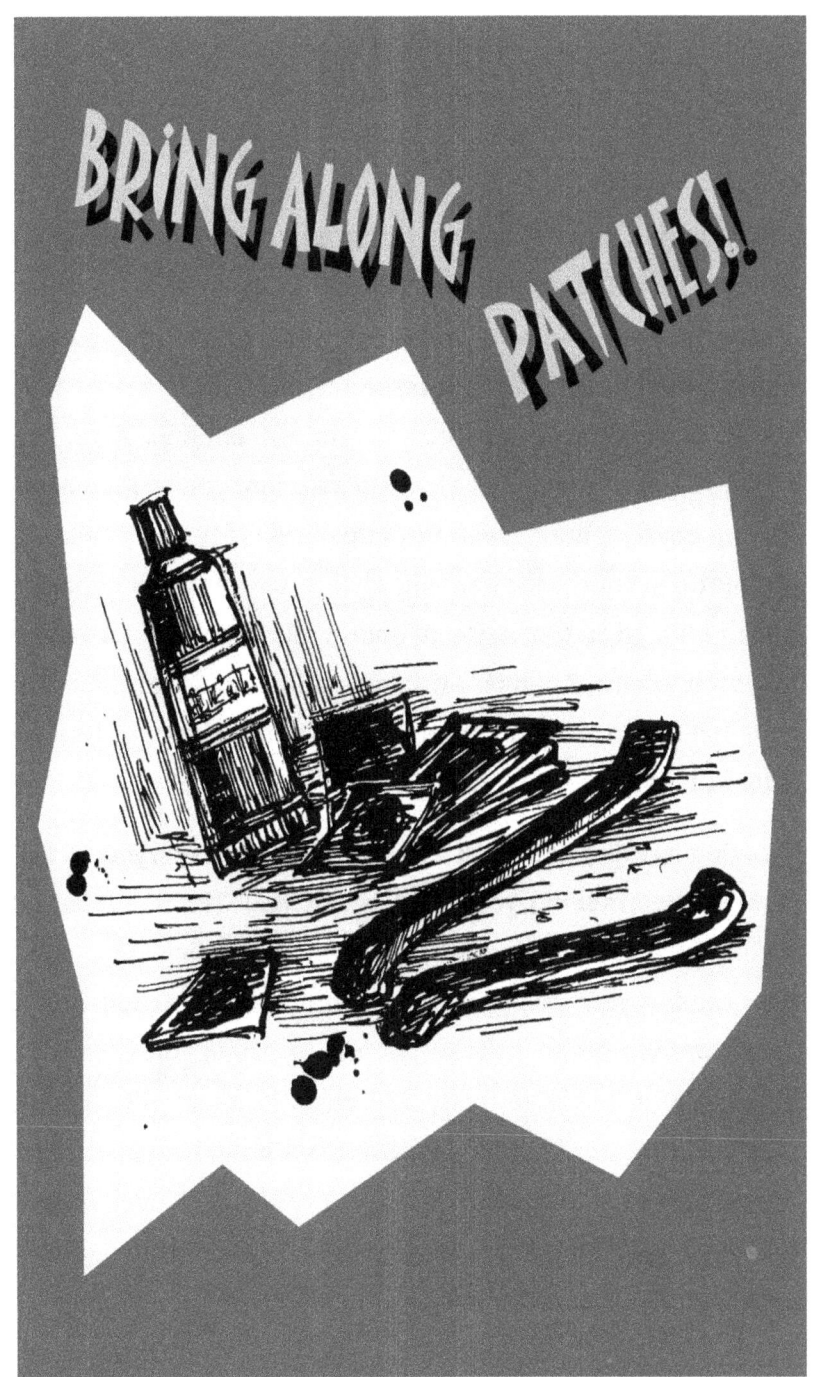

MONEY

You should have a wallet in your hydration pack. It should have at LEAST $10 cash inside ($20 is preferable), and not plastic money like credit cards. You never know when you are going to need something from a convenience store or food stand. Sometimes a nutrition bar is not enough. Also, you might see something cool at a yard sale that you have to have. Having cash on hand gives you added security and options in a situation. Your wallet should always be kept in a separate pouch clipped to the inside of your hydration pack. Or have a clip on it where it can be attached to the inside. In the event your hydration pack's zipper comes open, this will keep it from falling out.

Losing a wallet can work a person into a frenzy trying to find it, and backtracking your path is not fun. The likelihood of finding your wallet is remote, even in trail riding. That's the best reason your biking wallet should have no credit cards, debit cards, store gift cards or anything that will be distressful if lost. Keep only $20 cash, in small bills. Losing $20 is a lot better than having to deal with the hassle of a lost credit card or a debit card. And losing nothing is even better! So, keep your wallet secured to your pack! And for double measure, buy a cheap wallet.

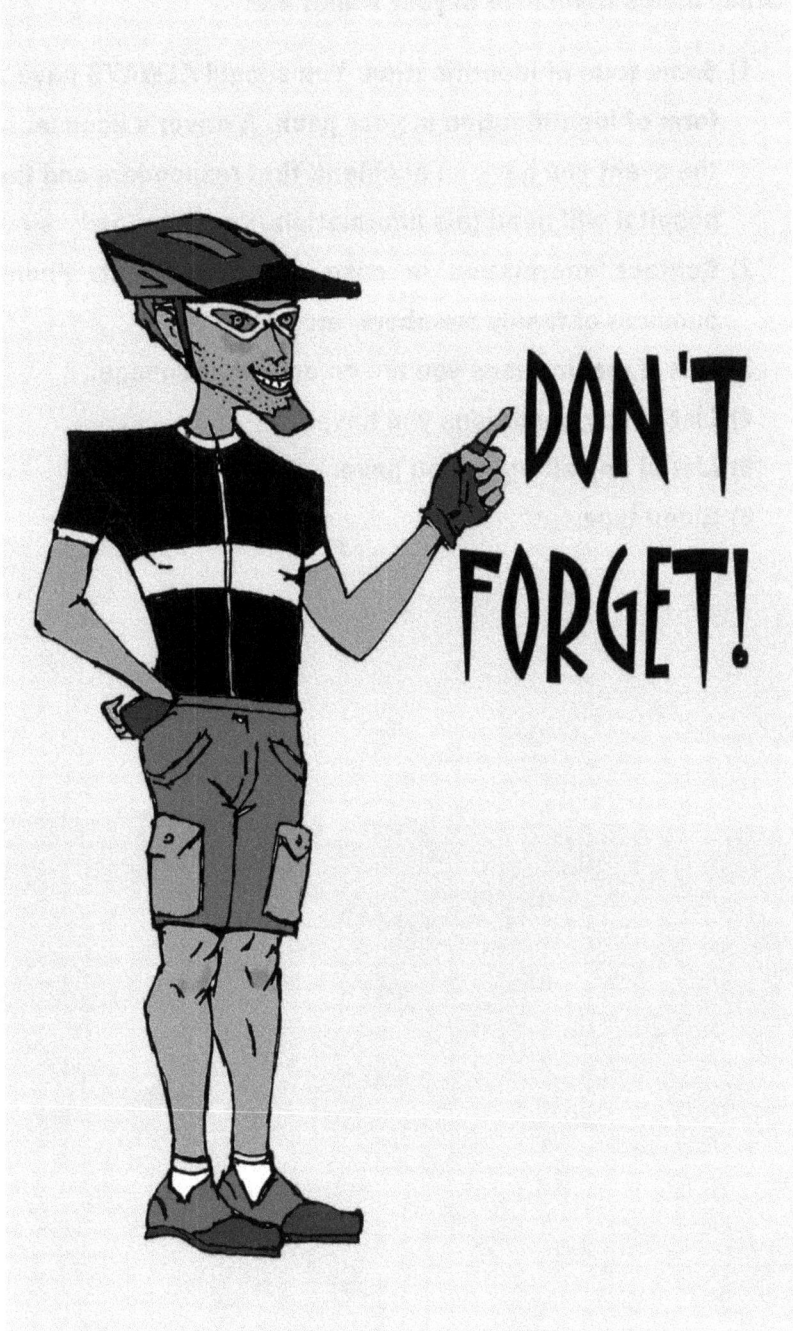

Other things to include in your wallet are:

1) Some form of identification. You should ALWAYS have a form of identification in your pack. A driver's license. In the event you have an accident, first responders and the hospital will need this information.
2) Contact information in case of an accident. Phone numbers of family members, etc.
3) List of medications you are on and what dosage.
4) List of any conditions you have.
5) List of any allergies you have.
6) Blood type.

MISCELLANEOUS

Miscellaneous things are anything you can think of that you might need on your ride. Your ride might be an all-day ride, so you will need other things, like a jacket, cap, or more money.

One important consideration is what to do with your keys. Keys are objects that need to be kept handy and safe from falling out of your pack and getting lost. I have a simple solution that has worked for me for years:

Things needed:

1) Detachable two ring keyring that can be separated between the rings.
2) 18-inch shoestring or keyring coil.

Here's what to do:

1) Simply unclip and separate the keyring in two. You will have one side with the keys and the other without keys.

2) Now take one end of the string and tie it to the lowest part of the shoulder strap. Right side if you are right-handed, left side if you are left-handed.

3) Tie the ring of the keyring (side with keys) to the end of the string.

4) Now connect the other ring of the keyring (side without keys) to the plastic strap-adjuster on the shoulder strap.

5) Now connect the keyring together. Unclip the keyring when keys are needed. Simple!

This can be done inverted, with your keys attached to the lowest part of the shoulder strap, to keep your keys out of the way. I find this works better than having keys on the upper torso. I have never had the string catch on anything while riding so far. This works great for me. See illustration.

NOTE 1: A plastic swivel eye snap hoop can be used instead of a detachable keyring. I find it easier to unfasten. You can use the loose loop from the string knot to attach the snap hook to.

NOTE 2: The keys connected to your hydration pack should be copies and not your usual keys. These stay with your pack. Also, limit the keys to only what you truly need. For example, a house, car and bike lock key.

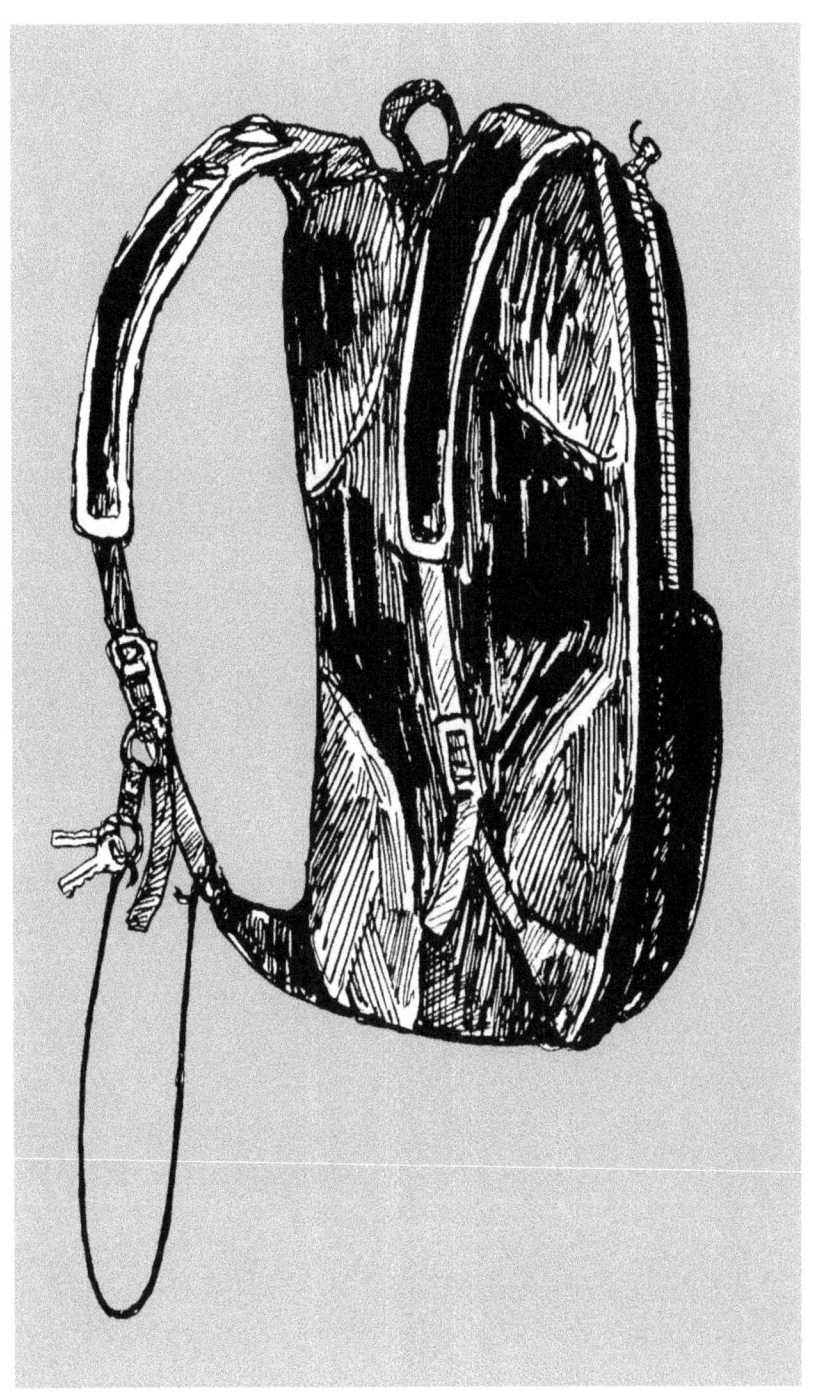

Pack Smart!

GEAR SMART - THE ART OF WHAT TO WEAR

HELMET/HEADWEAR

JACKET

JERSEY

SHORTS

UNDERGARMENTS

SHOES

SOCKS

GLOVES

GLASSES

HELMET/HEADWEAR

A rider should always wear a helmet. A helmet is first and foremost in cycle gear. Helmets are not heavy. They are made of foam and a thin plastic shell. Most these days come with a visor that keeps the sun out of your eyes, which I find to be indispensable. Newer helmets have an adjusting device that helps a person dial in their head size, creating a snug fit. They also have nylon straps and plastic locking clips that you clasp together under your chin.

When buying a helmet, always try it on first and look in a large mirror. Also look at your profile while wearing it. Why? Because some helmets are too oversized for the average head. Yes, the fit can be dialed in and made to fit all head sizes, but the actual helmet remains the same, too big! It's that same middle-ground approach to marketing, just like some manufacturers have for bike frames...one size for everyone! This issue, along with others, like a helmet that sits too high on the head, used to be notorious with department store helmets. And these issues still linger on in no-name brands today. But, happily, that is changing. Department stores now carry well-known brands that have age-specific fitting. Meaning, they are offering more sizes than one.

There's nothing wrong with going budget and buying a department store helmet, provided it fits good, looks good, and is a well-known name. To me, the protection it offers would be equivalent to any expensive helmet. The big brands in department stores are competitive and have the edge, providing the best in innovation and new design. You can't ask for more. So, do some shopping around and find one that fits.

In choosing a helmet, it's best to find a color that has some universal color-coordinating appeal, like black, white, silver, or gray. These colors will go with any cycle dress color or bike color. And lastly, be cautious of buying a helmet online unless you know exactly what you are buying. If there is no way to try it on, it's best to forgo the purchase, no matter how sporty it looks. Remember, a helmet should not look like you have a helmet perched on your head, but rather like you are wearing a helmet!

TIP 1 – Sometimes in cold weather you will need something to put under your helmet to keep your head and ears warm. A thin stretchable sport fleece beanie is perfect for the job. Today's sport beanies, while very thin, block the cold well and fit easily under the helmet. Some even have reflective graphics on them. At the end of the winter season, these are marked down at a low price at major department and retail stores. Since these can be expensive, especially for the good brands, it's a good idea to take advantage of these seasonal markdowns and stock up. Think ahead!

TIP 2 – You should be able to fit two fingers under the neck straps for the right amount of helmet tightness and comfort.

The strap adjusters (left and right) should be under the ears, and the straps should be flat against the head.

TIP 3 – Do not paint or add stickers to your helmet. This will void any warranty the helmet has.

TIP 4 – Replace your helmet after a hit to it. It is possible the helmet has been cracked or the foam has been compromised in some way (perhaps not visible) by the hit. It is also recommended by some that you replace your helmet every 3 years.

TIP 5 – Remember, bike helmets are required by law now (in California). Also, having a helmet does no good if you are not wearing it! Check your city and state laws concerning bicycle helmets.

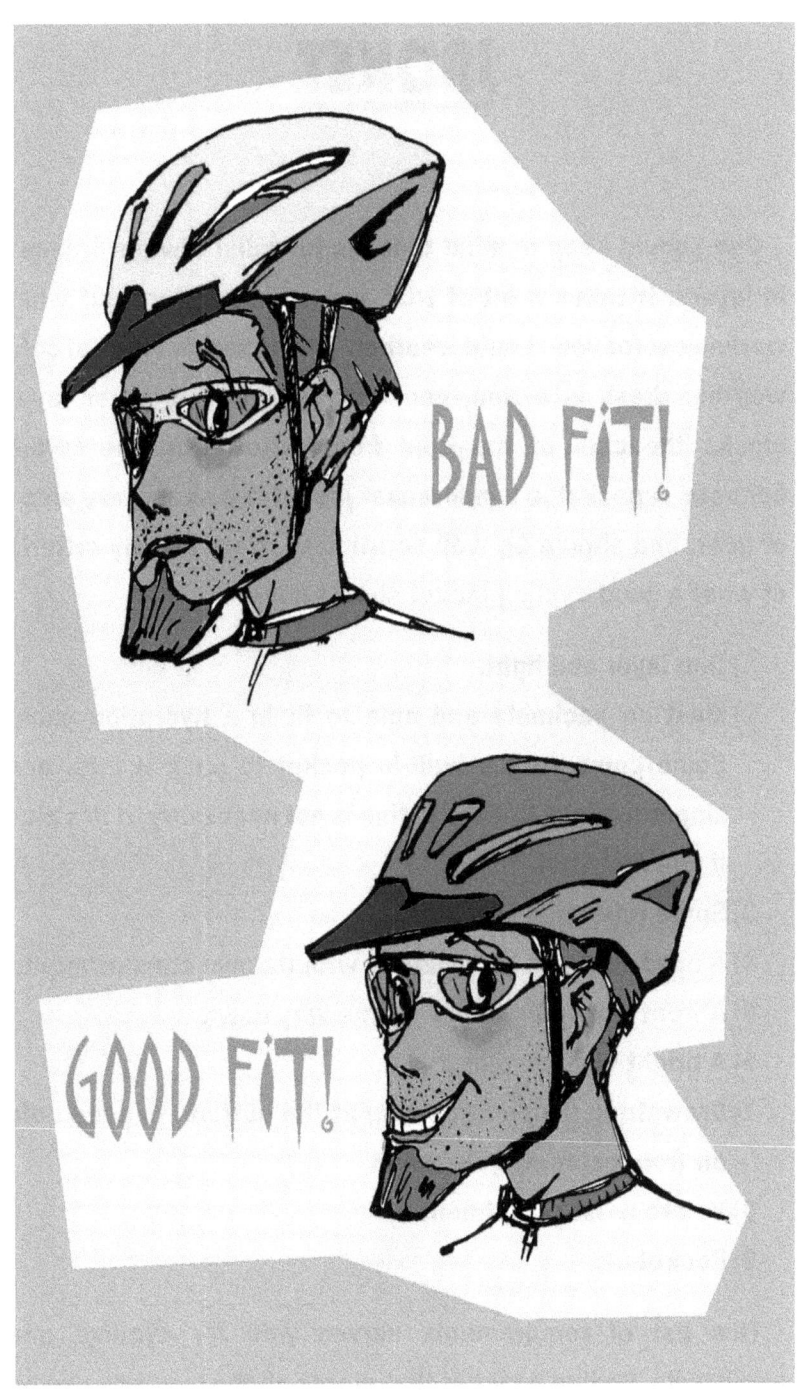

JACKET

One should keep in mind that the bicyclist always dresses in layers. It takes a bit of trial and error to figure out what works best for you in cold weather. The outermost part of cold weather dress is a thin, packable jacket. This outer layer blocks the chill of the cold from penetrating the layers beneath. A packable windbreaker jacket is a necessary piece of gear, and should be well scrutinized. Here are my criteria of what a good cycling jacket should have:

1) One layer and light.
2) Must be packable and able to fit in a hydration pack. Some come with a built-in pocket to pack it into, and zipper to close it (though this is not necessary, it is a plus if you find one).
3) Some reflective graphics.
4) A hood that can be rolled up with its own compartment.
5) A front zipper that goes all the way down.
6) A bright visible color.
7) Drawstring (nylon or cotton) at the bottom, to keep cold air from going up your waist.
8) Velcro wrist adjustments.
9) Pockets.

This list of requirements serves well for cycling, and admittedly, finding a jacket that meets all these needs can be quite a challenge. Also, because jackets are seasonal items, your quest for the perfect jacket becomes especially hard, but not impossible.

Start your search in a department store, and look for a one-layer, all-purpose sport jacket. An all-purpose sport jacket is usually low cost in comparison to a jacket made for cycling alone, which can be expensive. Actually, the difference physically between the two is minimal. They are made generally with the same materials and have very comparable features. Runners, joggers, and cyclists all have similar needs. So, I see no need to spend big. Going budget here is perfectly fine. And when you finally find one that meets these requirements, grab it! Maybe two! Be Gear Smart!

TIP 1 – If your jacket does not have a pouch built into it to store it, you can stuff it in a small ankle sport sock. This works for me. The main thing is to make it compact and packable.

TIP 2 – The waist drawstring must be a string, with no elastic. Wrist adjustments must be Velcro, with no elastic either. Following this will ensure longevity to your jacket. Elastic features have no durability in **ANY PART** of a jacket. Why? Because rubber/latex breaks down relatively quickly, even in storage. The polyester part of a jacket will last for a great many years. But the elastic features will deteriorate early, leaving the rest of the jacket useless. A jacket is only as good as the fastening parts. So, no elastic on any part of the jacket! If you follow this rule, your jacket will last for many years.

JERSEY

I don't know about you, but I like to dress appropriately for the sport I engage in. All sports have a uniform that is aimed for performance, function, identity, and team colors. Cycling is no different. The cycle jersey is a characteristic sport shirt designed for cycling. It is one that has not changed much through the years. It is thin, cool, and formfitting. It is also sporty and very colorful, often being embellished with logos of bike sponsors, brands, and graphics covering the entirety of the shirt.

Bicycle jerseys, by design being genuinely nice sport shirts, can be pricey, depending on whose name is on it and the quality. But I don't think one needs to overdo it here. After all, the everyday rider is not a pro rider sponsored by a bike company. So, why pretend? Here, some middle ground wisdom is in line. I find that there are lots of reasonably priced, good brands and fine quality bike jerseys that are sold online. There is no reason to go to a bike store and overspend.

These online jerseys come with an assortment of cool graphics, too. There are plenty whose images are "hip" and "stylish," and will not call you out as a cheap cyclist. Most, if not all, are made and shipped from overseas. The same can be said of most of the more expensive bike store bought jerseys.

Most jerseys are made in Asian countries with smaller framed men, making ordering the perfect fit problematic. You most likely have to order your jersey one size up, or even two. So, pay careful attention to the sizing guide the seller offers.

You certainly can look good as you ride, without having to shell out the big bucks.

Remember: It is better to ride a good bike and dress inexpensively, than to ride a cheap bike and dress expensively.

TIP – It is not absolutely necessary to wear a jersey for riding. There are plenty of stretchy form-fitting sport shirts with moisture wicking properties that are sold just about anywhere men's sport clothes are sold. These are very similar to a jersey, minus the zipper and back pockets. They are also made with nice colors and are comfortable. Some have reflective graphics too. And best of all, they are inexpensive. These are marked down at certain times and can be bought at an incredibly low price. So, keep your eyes peeled for some bargains.

NOTE: Some riders prefer a more organic feel to the way they dress. And that's okay. Bright colors and form-fitting clothes make them feel like they are sporting a superhero costume, or they are a neon sign, and they would rather just blend. So, a t-shirt and some shorts are their thing. You don't have to be locked into a pro-cycling image to feel legit. Wear what makes you feel comfortable. Be practical and real. But do wear a helmet and gloves.

SHORTS

Bike shorts are kind of a paradoxical item for men. Men want to be both fast and dressed right, but are not too keen on wearing restrictive (junk-squashing) spandex and having their man parts vaguely on display. An average baggy type short, on the other hand, would be more comfortable and modest and better for the job, even though it does not make one feel fast.

Thankfully, these days there are cycling-specific baggy shorts that can fill this description. These cycling shorts fit snug (in the right areas) and are sporty at the same time. To some they might be expensive. So, if you want to go on the cheap on this article of clothing, there is a solution. Try finding a multi-use short that is geared for general hiking, camping, cycling, and sport. These are found in common club card stores and are inexpensive. Find a size that is snugger than your usual fit if you want a more form fit.

The material these shorts are made of are usually stretchy and allow for movement. Yes, they will not have the inner padding cycling shorts have, so there is a concession. Most have zippered leg pockets for stuff, and some come with a nylon belt. They look good with all cycle jerseys, provided you buy them in black or charcoal gray, general colors that match everything. Visually, they are not much different from a generic cycling short. But, if you are particular and want a true cycling short, and if you don't mind the cost, go to a bike store and buy some. Cycling-specific shorts can also be purchased online at a lower price than bike stores, but the shipping cost usually cancels out the cost effectiveness.

You should explore the different options, other than typical spandex shorts, and the feeling associated with them—riding around in your underwear commando style!

NOTE: Do not dry any article of cycle gear in the high heat setting of your dryer. Follow the recommendations of the tag. Any clothing that has elastic will get ruined with high heat. The elastic waistband of spandex shorts will be ruined and no longer fit tightly around your waist.

UNDERGARMENTS

Cold weather undergarment dressing: I find the best cold weather undergarments to consist of a thermal shirt (long sleeve with crew neck) and a pair of cold weather stretch pants (thermal leggings).

Changing temperatures and chill factors dictate how you need to dress on any ride. This requires some considerable foresight, because warm undergarments can't simply be removed on the fly if the temperature warms up. Why? Because these garments are under all your other clothes, as is the case with a thermal shirt and pants (unless you want to give others a free show on the side of the road).

So, if it heats up, you are miserably overheated till you get home. This happens with early morning rides. It starts off cool, but the sun comes up and it gets hot quickly. Wearing a thermal shirt and thermal pants would be too much in this case. And on some days, it can stay cold, but not chilly, so you may need to forgo the thermal shirt and thermal pants here, too. Body heat will warm you up. Yet, on a cold and chilly day, you will stay cold due to the chill. Your body heat will not help much. So, here you absolutely will need a thermal shirt and thermal pants and a windbreaker jacket. It is advisable that you know what the weather forecast is before any ride.

Night Rides: On night rides, it will stay cold, so just dress appropriately for a stable low temp. I find, in riding in cold nights and cold days, the upper attire consisting of the following items is perfect in this order: First a thermal shirt, then a t-shirt, then a jersey, and lastly a thin jacket. Dressing in this logical order by layers is the way to dress for night and cold weather cycling. Shed as you heat up!

For cold weather lower attire: sport form-fitting stretch pants (leggings) are to be worn under your shorts and over briefs. These keep your legs warm and cold air from flowing under your shorts. I usually roll them up above the calf. However, these sport stretch pants (leggings) are not too thick, and are not fully adequate for very cold night rides. So, buy the fleece type, as this type blocks the harsh cold very well. This type I wear all the way down to the ankle. Keep both for varying temps as needed. It is best to purchase these—like beanies and other gear—at the end of season, for half price or more off. Stock up and be "Dress Smart!"

TIP 1 – Remember that morning cycling always presents an attire quandary, simply because calculating the heat factor can be tricky. Is it going to warm up or stay cold? Will my body heat warm me up enough? Will I overheat or freeze? So, what should I wear? Here, understanding the season helps most.

TIP 2 – Cycling clothes should be form-fitting. Besides looking sloppy, baggy jerseys, shorts, and jackets flap in the wind and slow you down. Although not much, still, there is a practical reason beyond the aesthetic reason to wear clothes that hug the bod.

TIP 3 – It is advisable to carry a thin, full-face thermal ski mask, or a sport scarf rolled in your hydration pack, when riding on very cold nights. Very chilly air can cause a feeling of breathlessness while riding, which can be a big problem. A rider will be forced to stop and frantically try to warm up his/her breath and may feel light-headed and as though his/her lungs are locking or freezing up. This can be distressing. The only option without a ski mask or scarf is to pull the front top of one's jacket above the mouth and nose and breathe into it. I've been in this situation before and it's not fun. I regretted not bringing a ski mask or scarf. Air temperature can drop very quickly on winter nights, especially if the skies are clear. Also, as a rider passes city zones to more natural areas, the difference in temperature can be profound. Areas with hills and brush are vastly colder than paved city regions, and this can be felt unmistakably as you ride from one area to another. A rider needs to understand this and plan for it in advance.

Ski masks and sport scarfs can be purchased on sale late in the winter season at department stores. Buy either, roll it in your hydration pack, and survive the freeze!

SHOES

    Your choice in shoes depends on if you have toeclips and straps on your pedals or clipless pedals. If you have toeclips and straps attached to your pedals, you can use any running or active type shoe. I would make sure that the shoe you use has some leather or extra material on the front part of it. Reason being, your large toe will push against the front of the toeclips, creating a hole in time if the front part of the shoe is lean on material. This is truer if your toeclips are made of metal rather than composite plastic. If you have clipless pedals, you are limited to using only shoes that are made for them.

TIP – Black, sport type shoes work well and match any clothing.

SOCKS

For most riding, "ankle socks" will work perfectly. They are the best of many lengths to choose from. And as far as graphics are concerned, they do not have to be designer socks with your bike's logo printed on them or anything fancy. A stripe or two will do. As far as color, white or black. These will match everything. Black socks do get a bit hot, whereas white are relatively cool. But black socks do look more cycle-trendy. If you would like some added protection to the mid-calf and shins, wear mid-calf socks or crew instead. These too get hot, but that's a small price to pay for a little more protection from a hit to the shin by the pedal.

TIP – Chain retail department stores carry a large selection of athletic socks, if you want to be more stylish. The choice of flashy colors and graphics abound. So, indulge yourself!

NOTE: Socks **CAN RUN SMALL**, especially around the ankle. So, check the ankle width and stretch before you buy.

GLOVES

These days you can buy reasonably priced cycling gloves in just about any department or retail clothing store. So, you can buy several pairs and keep them handy where you store your cycle gear. When buying, make sure they are designed for cycling, because cycling gloves have cycling-specific padding distributed where it is vital. Although, any sport workout glove will do the trick, if that's all you have. Better that, than nothing.

TIP – Wash your gloves often and hang them to dry. Gloves will begin to smell like a locker room if washing is neglected. They also will deteriorate quicker if not washed often.

NOTE 1: Riding with gloves is important. It feels better than bare hands, and helps with any numbness. And gloves keep your hands warm in the cold. Also, while riding, a rider might fall off their bike, which basically means that their hands will forcefully meet the rough dirty pavement or trail. Protect your hands. Wear gloves!

Note 2: Every few years, department store chains will drop a bike accessory company in favor of a different one. When they do this, they discount entire lines of bike products and supplies. It pays to visit the bicycle section from time to time for these great deals.

GLASSES

Glasses are a must when riding. Besides the logical reason of better visibility and eye protection from UV rays on a bright sunny day, glasses are needed to protect the eyes from any airborne insects and things that might be in the air. It is possible to be hit in the eye by a bee while riding. I have! Besides shaded sunglasses, it is also good to have an additional pair of clear glasses for night riding. Find some with UV protection, useful for sunsets, cloudy days, and daylight times where shaded glasses would be too dark.

Make sure your cycling glasses are the narrow type, on both your shaded and clear glasses. Reason being, if the glasses are too tall, they will dig into the ridge of the nose because they will be pressed down by your helmet. This can make a ride miserable. So, test the fit of your glasses with your helmet before a ride. And even better, test them before you buy them.

TIP 1 – Glasses should be worn under the straps of the helmet, not over them.

TIP 2 – It is a good idea to have straps for your glasses. While attempting to remove your glasses while riding, you may drop them on the road. This can scratch them and ruin them. So, keep them secure, use straps!

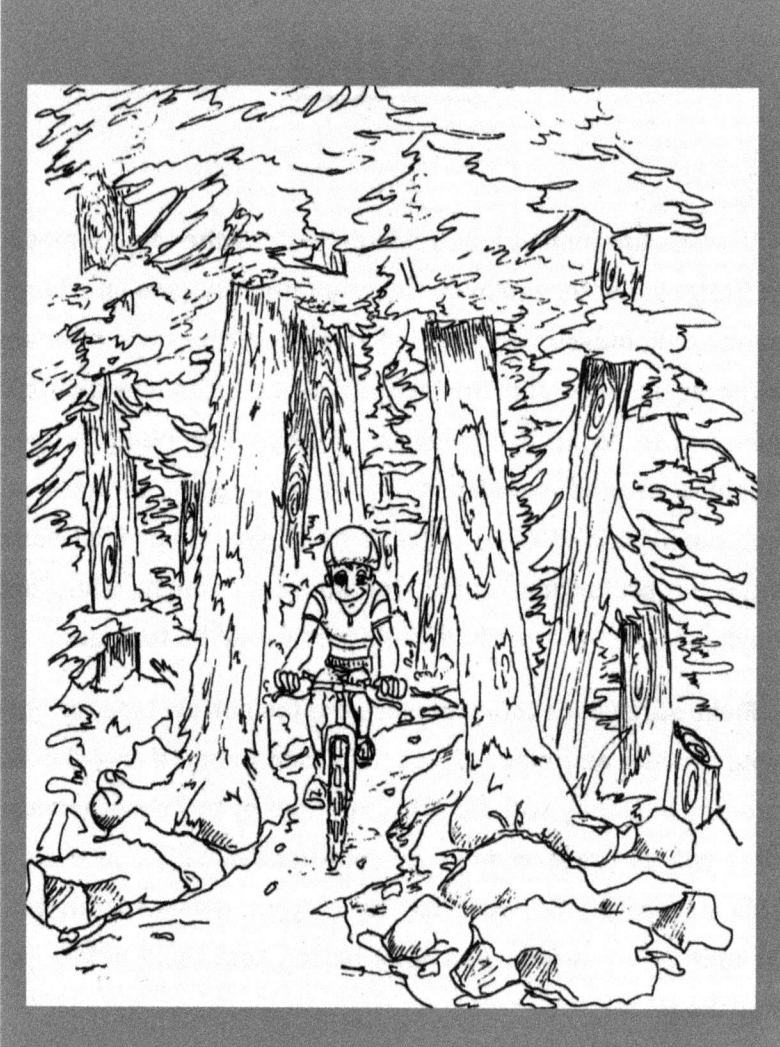

BIGFOOT COUNRTY

RIDE SMART - THE ART OF THE SAFE RIDE

THE SHAKEDOWN

VISIBILITY

CREEPS

CREAKS

THEFT

DOGS

TICKS

RIDE IN GROUPS

STRANGE ROAD HAZARDS

PROTOCOL AND HYGIENE

MASTER THE ROAD

NATURE CALLS

BIKE STORAGE

ONE WITH THE MACHINE

THE SHAKEDOWN

Even though this topic called "The Shakedown" might seem more logical to insert at the beginning of the book right after "Prepping," it can be a safety issue. So, it is appropriate to put here with the **ART OF THE SAFE RIDE**. Also, the beginner cyclist does not have the ability to **RECOGNIZE**, nor **KNOW-HOW** to deal with any bike issues. Inserting it in the beginning is putting the wagon before the horse.

Every bike goes through a shakedown period. The new bike shakedown is a time of testing your bike simply by riding it. In this period, a bike is given the royal run-through and a rider becomes acquainted with his/her new bike. In the process, there may be additional cable adjusting, brake pad aligning, and bolt tightening. All these come into play several months after the bike was originally properly built and tuned. There is nothing wrong with your bike, it's not falling apart. It's just being broken in. There are a lot of moving parts that can get loose. Additionally, along with further tunings, it becomes very clear to the rider what needs to be tweaked to tailor fit his/her bike more precisely. This is especially true of saddle height and saddle positioning. Also issues with stem height and length, and handlebar width.

This normal break-in phase helps to get the bugs out of your bike. After you complete all the things that need to be done, you will feel more comfortable and confident with your bike. At this point, you should not settle with anything that does not feel quite right. Small adjustments go a long way toward the feel of a bike and its performance. And that goes for just about everything on a bike. So, see it as a good thing and don't get too flustered. All bikes need a shakedown, even the pricey ones!

NOTE 1: Be sure to give your bike a pre-ride inspection before each ride. Check the tire pressure of each tire and inflate to the desired PSI. Confirm the brakes are working properly and that the pads are free of hard embedded debris. Check the quick release wheel levers to see if they are secure. Give your tires a quick look over for thorns and the like.

NOTE 2: Remember that the cheaper the bike, the longer it will take to get the bugs out of it. So, be patient, as it can be frustrating.

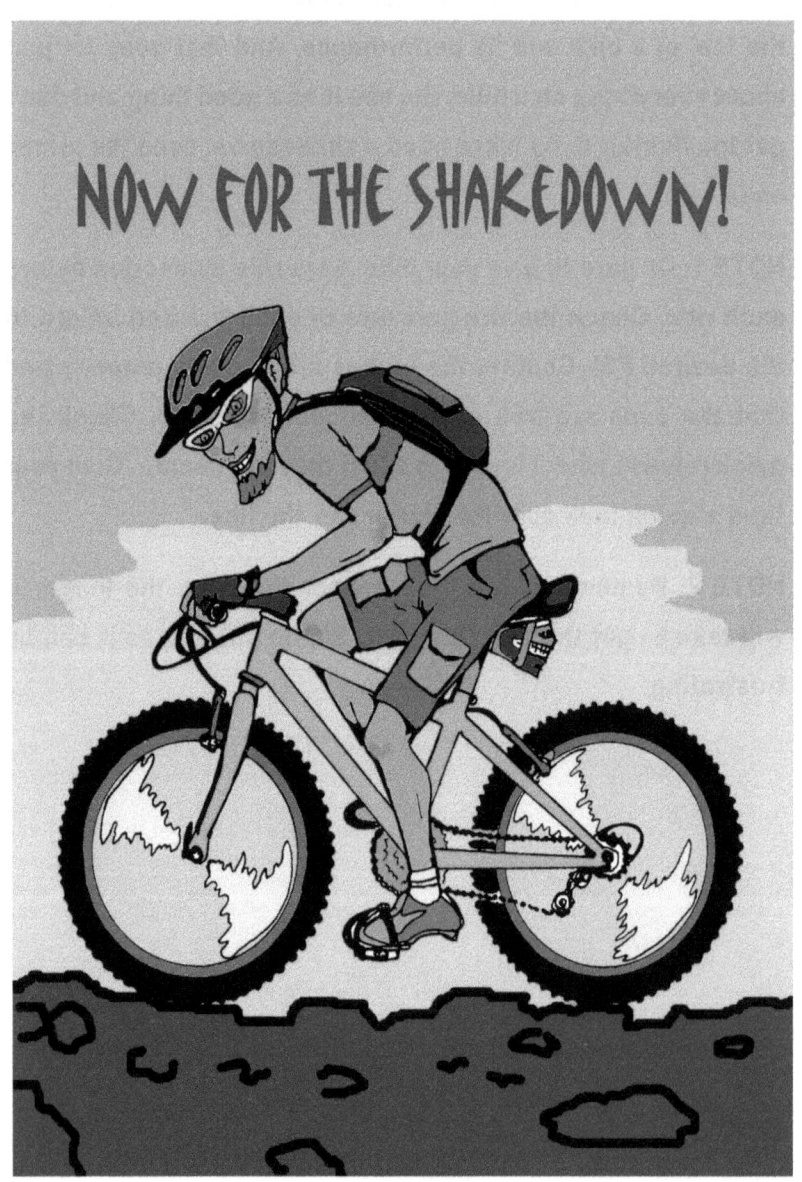

VISIBILITY

Never assume that people in vehicles see you. In fact, assume that they don't. So, do what you can to make yourself visible. It is wise to make eye contact with a person in a car who is waiting at the stoplight before you attempt to cross the crosswalk. This assures that they see you. Drivers are typically too preoccupied with traffic to consider cyclists.

Cyclists are hardest to see just after sundown. The twilight tends to confuse the driver's senses. Reason being, the sun has been at horizon level (eye level) for some time, and the eyes of the drivers have been driving in its glare. Now, the sun has just dropped below the horizon, and their eyes need to readjust from intense light to darkness. As a result, the light may seem brighter and the dark darker. Now, the driver needs to contend with all the moving bright vehicle lights and contrasting dark silhouettes in their field of vision. Between this light and dark, a cyclist can be hidden from sight within a dark shadow very easily.

So, as the sun begins to set, turn on your blinking lights and main light. Your night riding attire should be bright too. Black or dark colors are never a good idea for night riding.

TIP – Your night riding attire should be as bright and reflective as possible.

CREEPS

Be aware of your surroundings and any strange people around you. Also, look out for cars that seem to be tailing you or that are slowing as they near you, especially on secluded streets. Trails also have no shortage of weirdos and creeps that occupy them. I've seen strange people disappear into the bushes of local trails on several occasions, and people sleeping on the paved part of the trail. I've also passed up a person on a city trail only to see that same person about two blocks up the road as I passed him again, "Whaaaat?!" Strange, right?

Some protection is advisable and prudent. I think cyclists should carry pepper spray. They should keep it on their person or attached to their bike for easy access. A clueless cyclist is an easy target. SO, BE AWARE OF YOUR SURROUNDINGS AND be ALERT of PERSONS WHO ARE NEARBY!

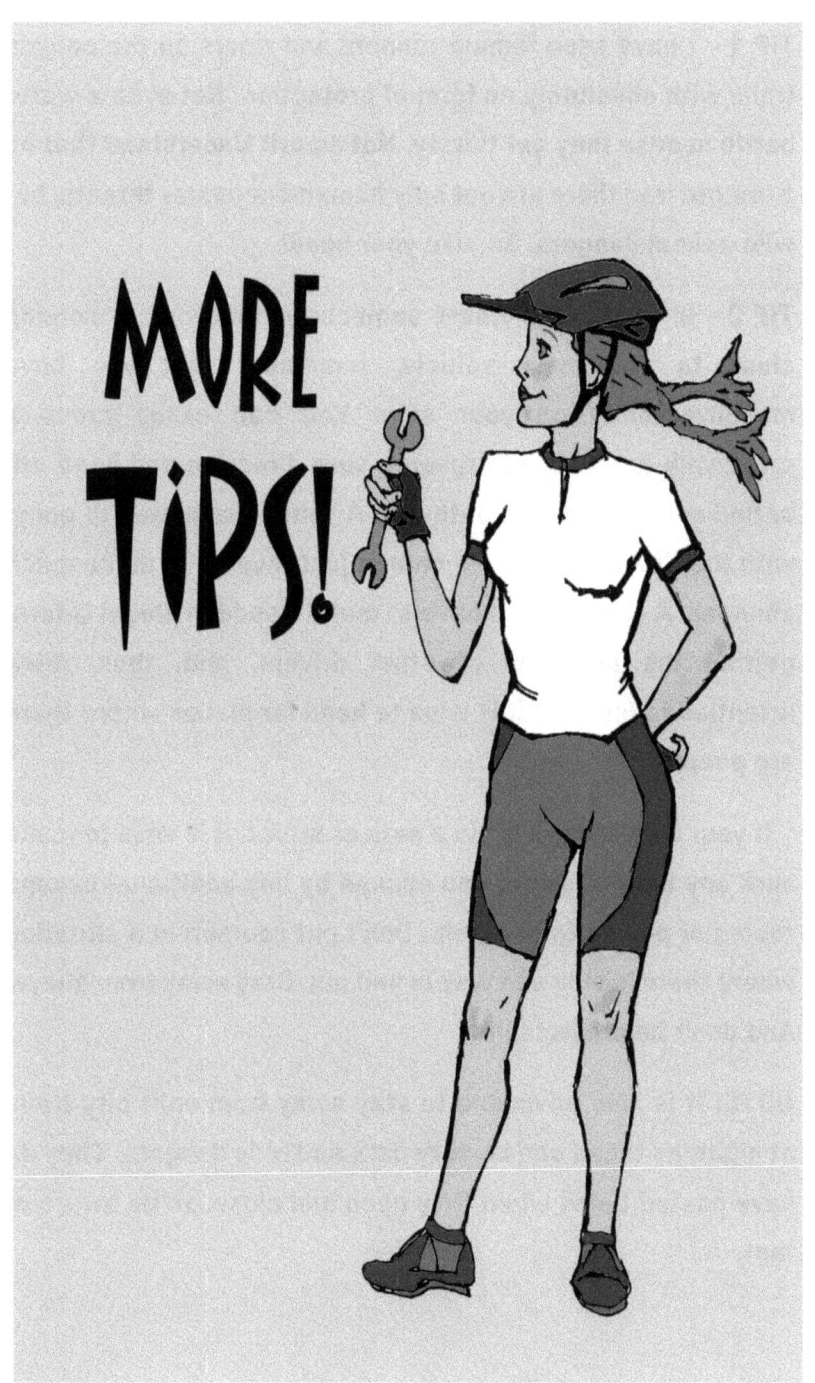

TIP 1 – I have seen female runners and riders on the canyon trails with absolutely no form of protection. Not even a water bottle in case they get thirsty. Not smart! Understand that on a remote trail there are not only human-encounter threats, but wild animal dangers. So, use your head!

TIP 2 – In a situation where someone is following or coming close to you in a vehicle, remember that you have maneuverability on your side. You can easily cross a crosswalk and turn and reverse your direction and head off, or find escape in a thin pathway. A vehicle is limited to going with the flow of traffic and cannot just reverse or make quick changes. A creep would have to make a sudden illegal U-turn, getting the attention of other drivers, and, thus, draw attention to himself. It is wise to head for places where there are people.

If your only escape is via a path or street, it is wise to make sure any path or street you escape by has additional escape routes or places to find help. Don't put yourself in a situation where there is only one way in and out. Stay away from alleys. And don't be predictable.

NOTE: It is also advisable to stay away from unlit city trails at night, as these can be very dark and hide dangers. They do have posted times when they open and close, so be aware of that.

TOPIC OF CONTENTION

Here is an item of contention that fits somewhat in the Creep category:

INVISIBLE WALKERS

At night, I see the vast majority of people on the trails (which are not lit) failing to wear proper colored clothing, and without some sort of light to make their presence known. I see them dressed in black or dark colors, running, walking dogs, or strolling children in the middle of the dark path. These people, their pets, the leashes, and the strollers are virtually invisible until you get very close. So, even a cyclist with a good bike light can barely see them—they just blend into the darkness. And given the average speed of a bike (11 to 14 mph), it is difficult to react in time to avoid a collision. In the case of such a collision, there will no doubt be a heated confrontation on the path, and possibly a legal nightmare afterwards. So, to the cyclist I say, "BE KEENLY AWARE OF ILL-PREPARED PERSONS ON THE TRAILS AT NIGHT OR NIGHTFALL. ALSO USE A BRIGHT HEADLIGHT. AVOID A COLLISION!"

CREAKS

I don't know about you, but a creaking bike drives me crazy. Creaks, pings, rattling, and ticking sounds are a giveaway that something is not right, or is loose on a bike. There are many kinds of irritating sounds a bike can make.

They're usually heard only when you are riding. Obviously! Normally, a bike should not make any sound when you ride it, except for the spinning tires and the sound of the freewheel doing its thing. So, you must play bike detective to find the source. If a bike just starts making a strange sound, consider any repair or adjustment you did last. That might be a clue.

Try to carefully home-in on the area of the sound. Does the sound happen as you pedal, or only as you coast? Do you hear it only if you are sitting on the saddle? Maybe when your hands are pushing down on the handlebars or while turning? In time, you will be able to identify the source just by the sound, and know exactly what the problem is. But here are some common areas of problem bike sounds and how to fix them:

1) Tick or creak sound as you put some weight on the handlebars. The problem(s): The handlebars are not centered in the stem, and/or the stem bolts are not tightened correctly or evenly. Solution: Correctly reposition handlebars in the

stem. Then retighten the bolts with small turns, alternating until each bolt is tight. Make sure the spacing between the clamp is the same from top to bottom. Another possible problem is that the stem bolts are too dry. Solution: Unscrew stem bolts, clean and lightly grease, then reinstall handlebars and tighten bolts. Make sure in either case that the area of the bars that is clamped by the stem is clean.

2) Rattling sound as you ride. The problem: The water bottles are hitting the frame or vibrating in the cages. Solution: Move anything that is hitting against the frame. Bend the cages to tighten their grip on the bottle.

3) Rattle, creaking, or buzzing sound as you pedal, heard near the water bottle cage. The problem: The water bottle cage bolts are loose. Solution: Tighten bolts and inspect the bosses.

4) A ticking sound as your crankarm reaches a certain position. The problem: The pedal bearings are dry or bad. Solution: Grease or replace pedal bearings.

5) A sharp deep ping sound as you pedal (usually also felt throughout the frame). The problem: The bottom bracket retainer is getting loose. Solution: Retighten it. You may have to use some Teflon tape on the retainer threads.

6) A sharp creaking sound near the chainrings as you pedal. The problem: A crankarm might be getting loose. Check the crankarms and see if there is any play (looseness). Listen for

that sound as you put some pressure on each arm. Check the bolts. Solution: Retighten bolt/bolts.

7) A chirping sound to the rear of your bike as you ride. The problem: The rear derailleur pulleys (jockey wheels) are dry and may be caked with crud. Solution: Clean and lubricate pulleys.

8) A scraping sound when the cranks are in motion. The problem: The front derailleur cage is contacting the moving chain. Solution: Adjust the front derailleur "H" limit screw, and/or add tension to the cable. You can also adjust the derailleur position (toe-in a bit).

9) Shifting chain sound in the front or rear derailleur while riding. The problem: The wrong cable tension is causing the chain to partially shift while riding. Solution: Adjust the cable tension.

10) A dull scraping or thumping sound near one wheel while riding. The problem: A brake pad is contacting the spinning rim. Solution: Center the wheel. Also, sometimes the brake cable casing is pushing on one brake arm, causing both to lean. Pull on the cable and straighten it. If the scraping sound continues, loosen brake cable tension enough to silence it.

11) A creaking sound while riding in a sitting position. The problem: The seat clamp bolts, seatpost (the part that is inside the frame), or saddle rails are overly dry. Solution: Lightly grease clamp bolts. Lightly grease seatpost (the part

that goes inside the frame). Lightly oil area between the clamp and seat rails.

12) A chattering and rattling sound is heard coming from the rigid fork or suspension (applicable to quill stem bikes) fork area as you go downhill, and especially when you use the front brake. The problem: The headset is coming loose. Solution: Retighten the locknut. Make sure you're not overtightening the headset and the steering is easy.

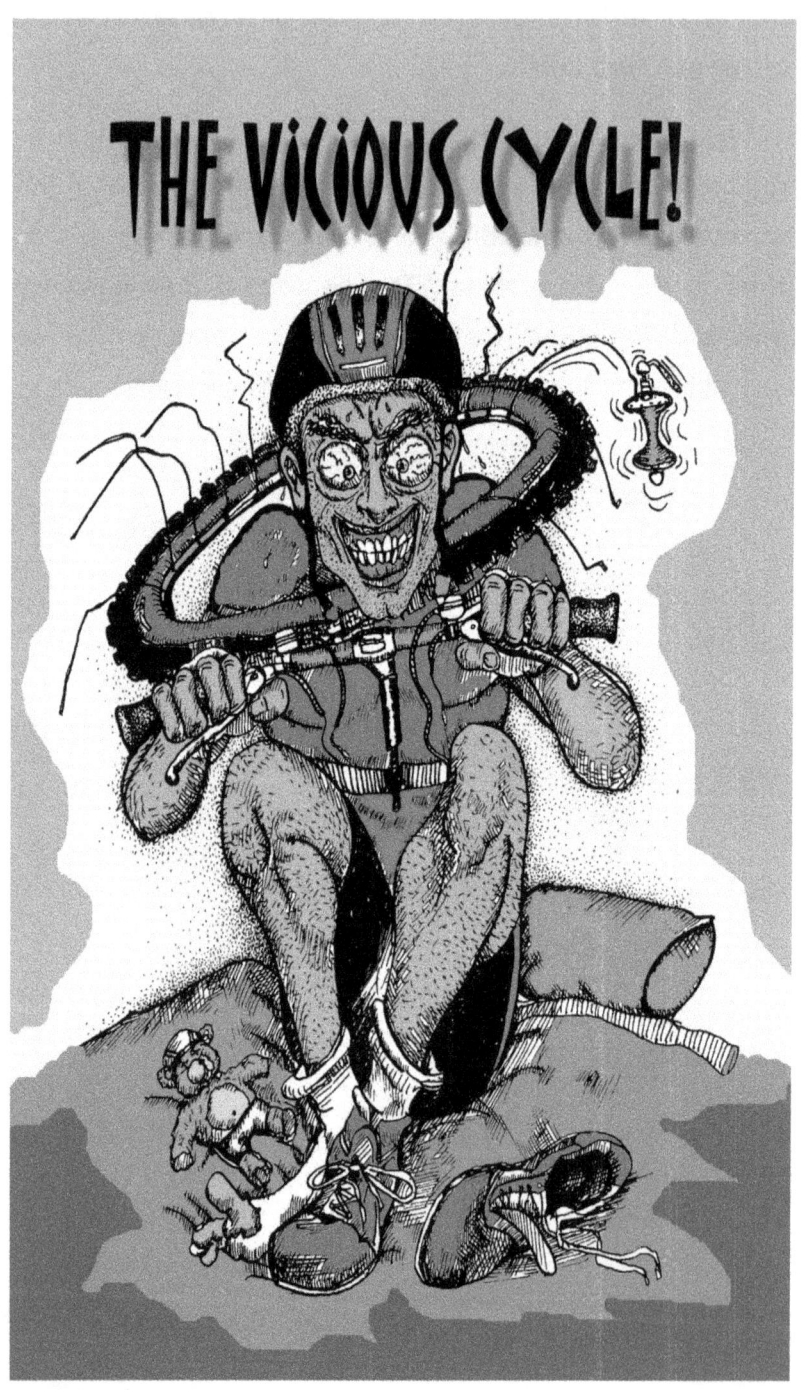

THEFT

If you ride a nice bike, assume a thief wants to steal it. It's all about resale. A bike thief is not looking to ride around on a stolen bike. He just wants to sell it quick and move on to the next bike theft opportunity. And understand, once a bike has been stolen, it is gone! **YOU WILL NEVER SEE YOUR BIKE AGAIN! IT'S A BIG WORLD!** So, if you stop to stretch on the trail, do not go far from your bike, and take notice of your surroundings. A thief in the brush can easily jump out, hop on your ride, and quickly pedal off.

Bike theft is becoming more sophisticated, and now bike thieves tend to work in pairs. One thief will try to distract you and get you off guard. And then the other will steal your bike. So, be wary if someone is trying to make small talk, even if he is **WEARING CYCLING GEAR AND HAS AN EXPENSIVE BIKE**. This is a ploy meant to evoke a feeling of camaraderie and trust—taking a rider by total surprise.

Eventually the crook will get you to stop and get off your bike. Then he or she will divert your attention while the partner comes along and grabs your bike. Then both, ride off into the sunset while you stand with your mouth open, thinking, "What happened?!" **BE AWARE** of theft ploys...Be also cautious of a pretty damsel in distress in the middle of a trail. This can be another ploy to make a rider stop.

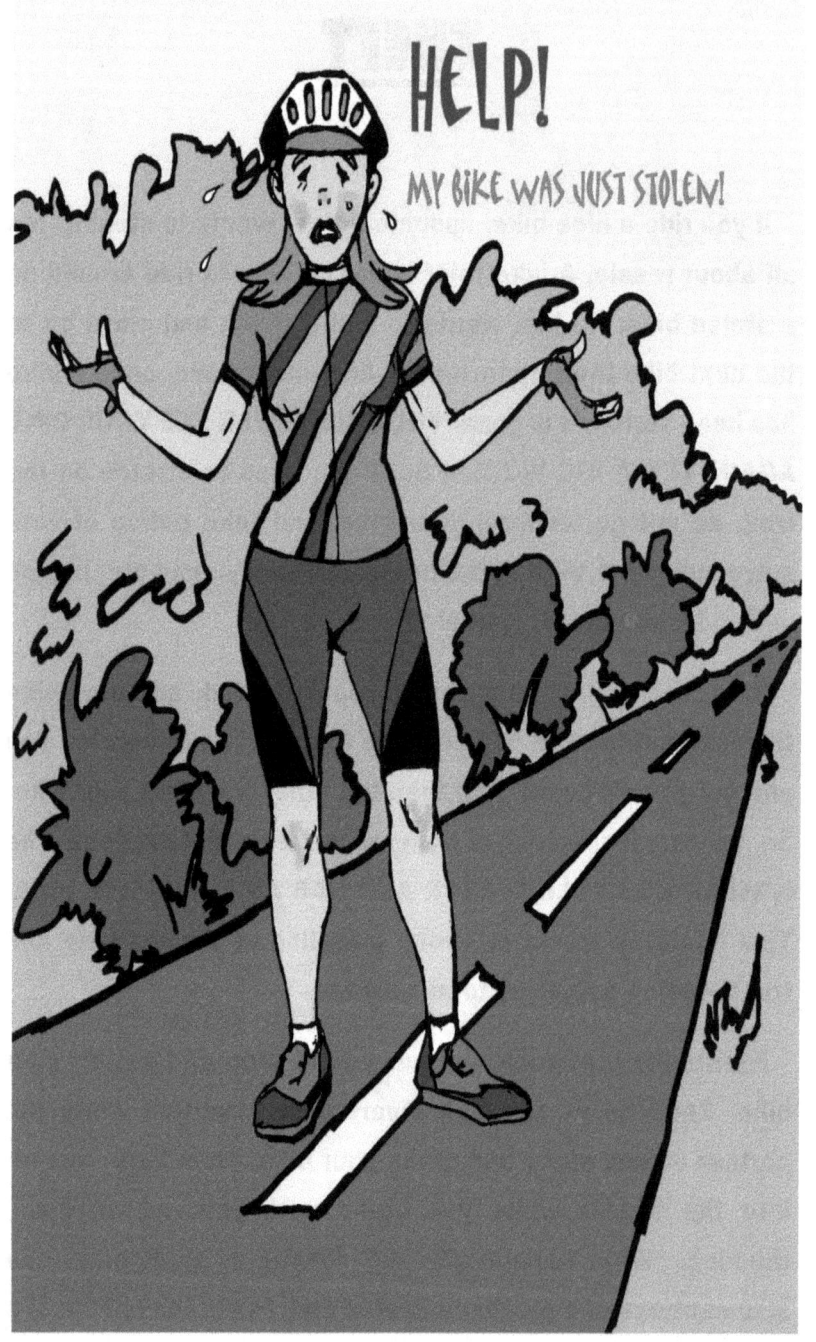

LOCKS

Realize that ALL bike locks, cables and the likes, can be broken into or cut. If a thief has the right tools for the job, it can be done quite easily and quickly. So, in reality, a bike lock is only a deterrent at best. If you are going to lock an expensive bike, **MAKE SURE THAT IT IS ALWAYS IN YOUR SIGHT.** If not possible, lock it in an area that has some sort of surveillance. But, even then, a person in a hoodie can steal your bike without having his or her face seen. Understand that bystanders are not going to confront, stop, chase-down, or detain a bicycle thief, or any thief for that matter. In fact, they will more than likely not want to get involved at all. So, it is best to keep your costly bike with you or not take it out for purposes other than sport. But there is a solution.

Some people have a "junker bike." A "junker bike" is a sacrificial bike that has had its day in the sun and that no one in their right mind would steal. People use their "junker bike" for going to the store and running errands. Some thieves will even steal a "junker bike" if they can make a buck from it. But at least it will not hurt as badly when it is stolen. And that's the point. So, the bottom line is, you cannot trust a lock for the protection of your bike, and you may have to resort to riding a junker.

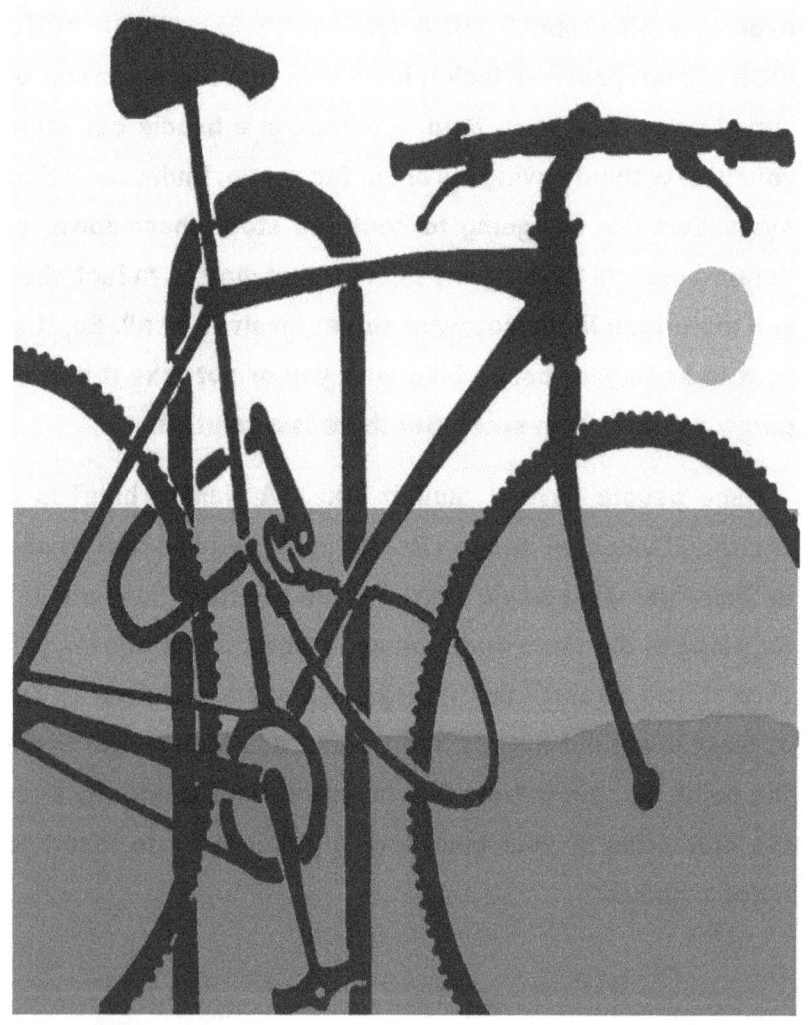

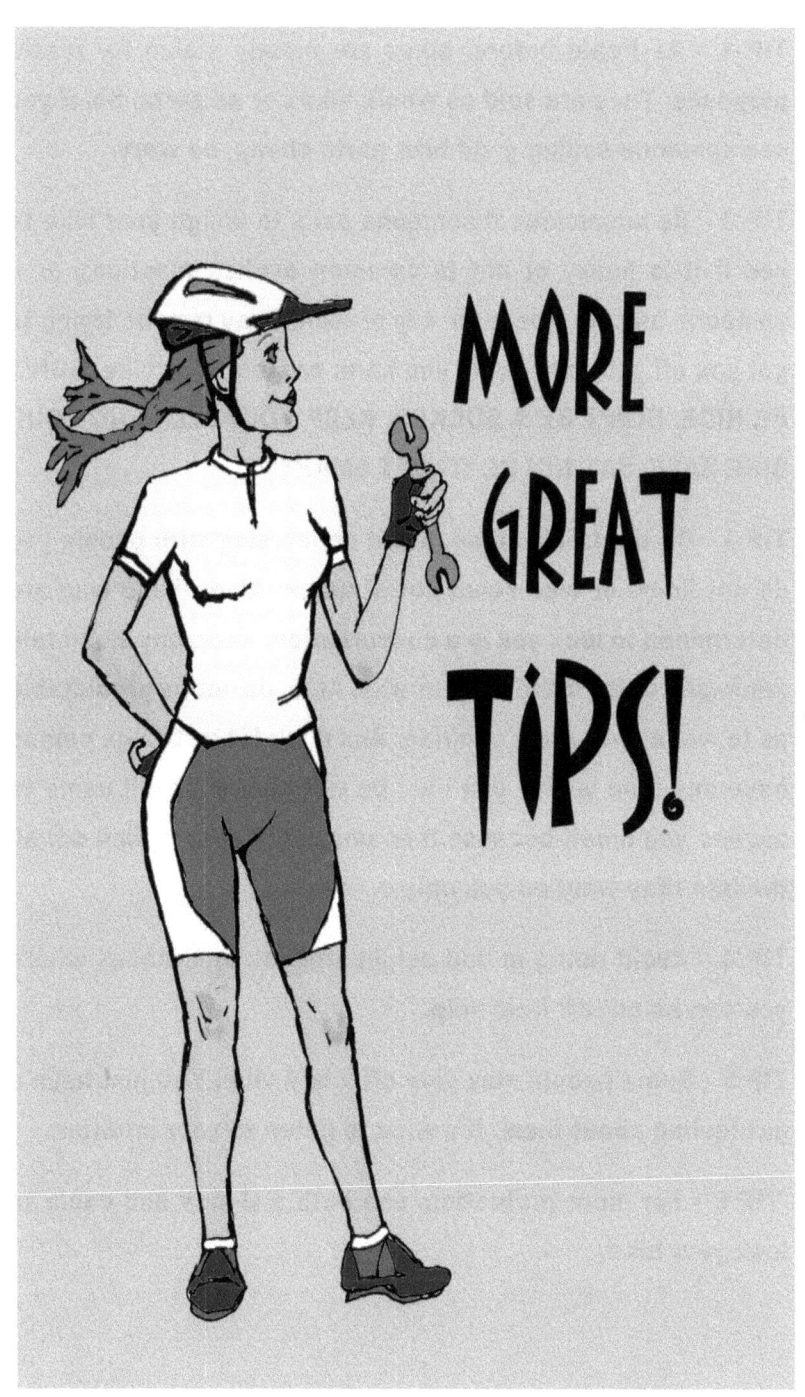

TIP 1 – As I said before, bikes are mostly stolen for resale purposes. They are sold as whole bikes or as parts. So, if you see someone selling good bike parts cheap, be wary.

TIP 2 – Be suspicious if someone asks to weigh your bike to see if it is heavy or not (a common cyclist question), or if someone asks to ride it for any reason. They may be trying to get you off your bike to do you harm or steal your bike. DON'T BE NICE. DON'T BE A SUCKER. KEEP YOURSELF AND YOUR BIKE SAFE. SAY NO! BE "THEFT SMART!"

TIP 3 – On the trail or road, avoid conversing with people you do not know or who seem out of place. Also, those who are determined to lock you in a conversation. Keep any small talk minimal, cut it off and go your way. Also, do not be predictable as to when and where you ride. And don't let a strange person have any idea where you live. Do not give your full name to anyone you meet, because it is amazingly easy to find out all the info they want on you online.

TIP 4 – Avoid riding in bad neighborhoods and places where you can be cut off from help.

TIP 5 – Some people may give off a bad vibe. You just have a gut feeling about them. It's wise to listen to your intuition.

TIP 6 – For more protection, use both a U-lock and cable to lock your bike.

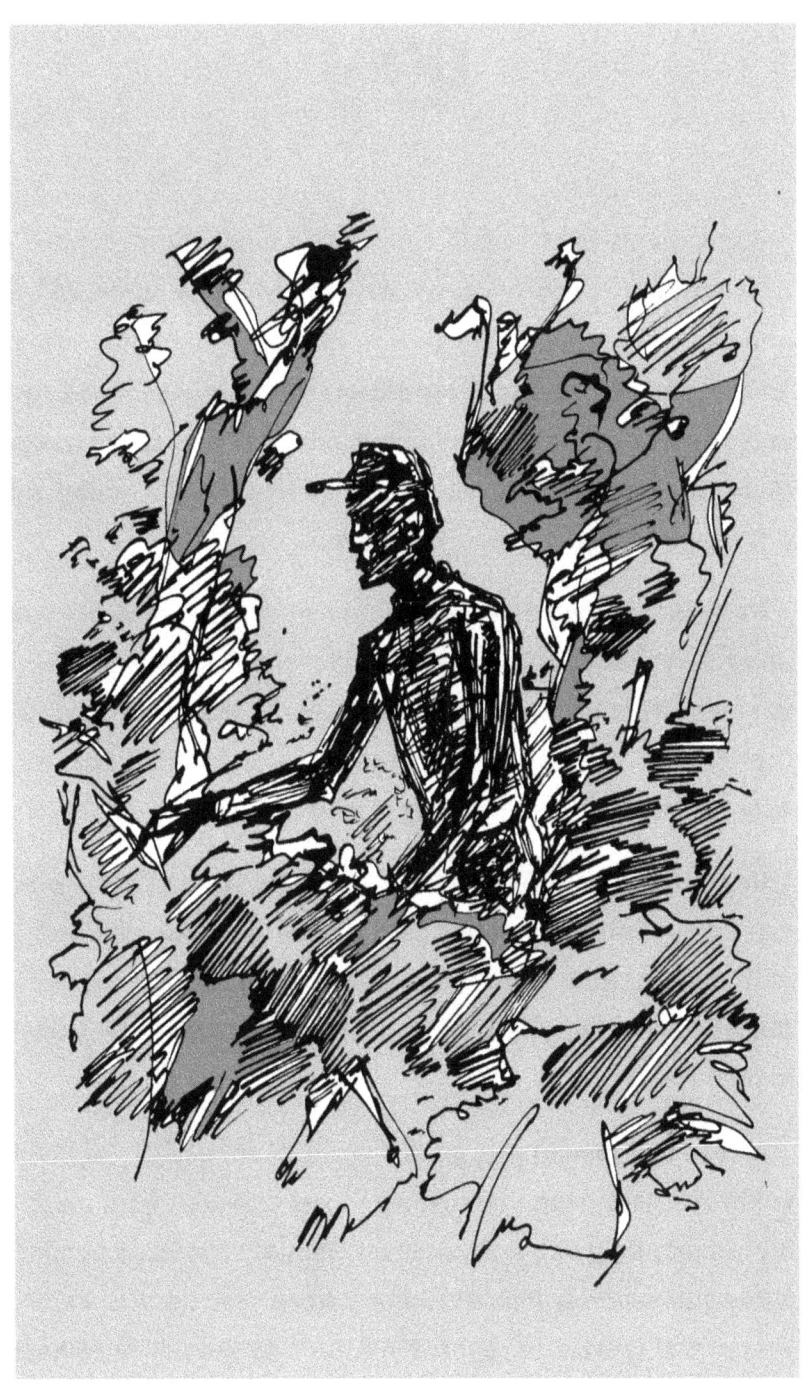

DOGS

Dogs, man's best friends, are not necessarily a bicyclist's best friend. Loose dogs are usually encountered in neighborhood areas. This is true in good neighborhoods as well as bad. It's best to avoid streets within blocks if you can, and stick to the main roads. A cyclist is seen as a strange thing to a dog and not recognized as friendly. So, a dog will often go after the person on the bike.

Here is an occasion where pepper spray might become necessary. Put your bike between you and the dog if you can't get away from the dog soon enough. Spray the dog with water first to see if he loses interest in you. If he continues the aggression, then pepper spray is your only resort.

Use wisdom here. Try a short spurt to let the dog know what can be expected if he continues. If that fails, let him have it with a direct short spurt; don't soak the dog. I do not savor the idea of spraying a dog. They are just doing what they think is their job.

Also, a dog cannot just go and wash its face after, so it will suffer if it gets pepper spray in its eyes and mouth for quite a bit of time. Only use it if you must. But, always keep in mind, a dog can severely injure or kill a human. You have to defend yourself. It is wise to report the attack to the police to keep it from happening to someone else, and to protect yourself from any retaliation or legal problems from the owner. So, the bottom line here is to avoid dogs as best you can. Be "Dog Smart!"

TIP 1 – Avoid eye contact with dogs. They see that as a threat. Just pretend you don't see them.

TIP 2 – If you are going to outrun the dog, and do so, make sure you have left him far behind you. Look back several times, because sometimes the dog is still in pursuit. That is possible. I know from personal experience.

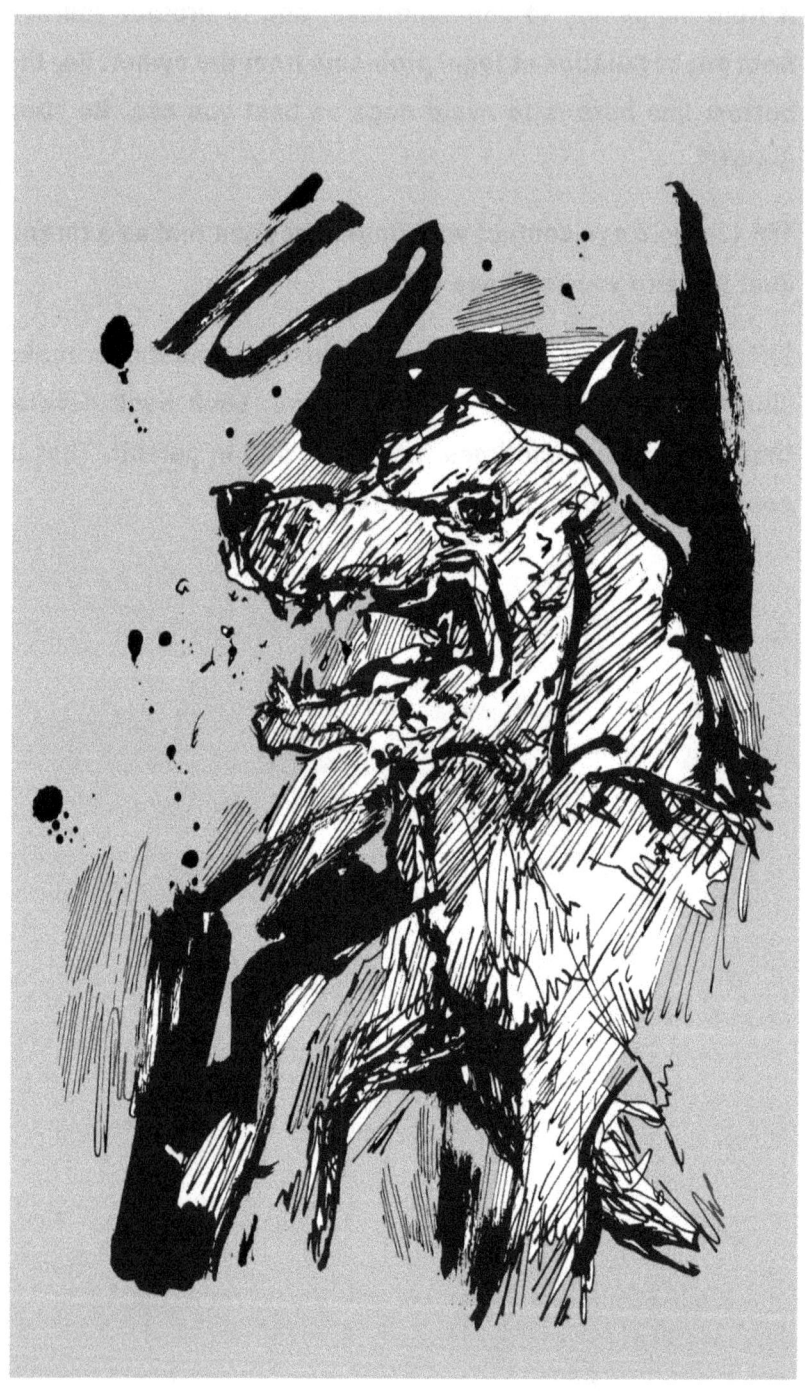

TICKS

If you are an avid mountain biker and love to explore new trails and byways, you should continually be on the lookout for ticks. Ticks are tiny crablike looking insects that have the potential to cause Lyme disease, a lifelong, even fatal, illness. It is something you do not want! Ticks can reside pretty much all over the trail, but especially in bushes and hanging branches, just waiting for an unsuspecting animal or person to drop on for its blood feast.

In the process of feeding, they can infect a person with the crippling disease. Not every tick carries the disease, but assume that they do. It's best to wear light clothing on the trail, socks especially. Light clothing will allow you to detect a tick more easily. Avoid contact with brush and branches and do not stand in one area for a prolonged time.

I took in the view at a scenic trail and stood for about 5 minutes at a dusty cliff side. Later, as I got home, I noticed a tiny bug crawling on my leg. Upon closer inspection, it was a tick! First time I encountered one. Luckily, it was not dining on me. So, shake off dirt and dust and do a quick tick check at the exit of the trail before you get home. And, when you get home, put your clothes immediately in the wash, and shoes and hydration pack outside for the night. Then check your body in the shower.

Also, you might want to keep a tick-removing tool in your pack and learn the basics of removal, for there are many different ways. Remember, if removal is done incorrectly, it could **GREATLY** increase the chance of being infected if the tick is carrying the disease.

And, if you do find one feeding on you, it's best to remove it the right way, or as soon as possible. Put it in a jar for reference, and see a doctor. Better safe than sorry. Lyme disease can be treated if caught early. Keep an eye out for strange bullseye-like rashes on your body, or any rashes for that matter. Always be mindful that on the trail, you are in tick country.

RIDE IN GROUPS

Cyclists are a community of people that share a common passion for biking. In your travels, you will no doubt come across fellow cyclists and befriend them. Of course, most riders on a pathway just want to get in their workout and be left alone—as is the case of people at a gym. But I do think it is important to get to know people who share the same trails and to become familiar with them, at least as acquaintances. Some of these acquaintances might even become "cycle buddies," and real friends down the road. Friends at your work, school or church can become "cycle buddies" or come together and form a weekend cycle group.

You have heard there is power in numbers, and that is true. A group of cyclists are easily seen and are taken more seriously than a single cyclist. So, there is some security found in not riding alone. Also, having conversations on a ride will help you to not focus so much on the miles ahead. And you'll be surprised that the length and difficulty of a trip will seem less so when shared with a friend.

When choosing a "cycle buddy," it is wise to make sure this person is at the same level of fitness as you are and has a similar bike with the same specs as yours, especially the gear ratios and wheel size. Otherwise, you'll suffer the frustration of having to wait, while they catch up to you. Or maybe, you'll be the one having to catch up to them!

TIP 1 – A group of cyclists usually have breakfast after a long ride. This can be a good social event and help you to meet other cyclists in the group. Meeting other cyclists can increase your social circle as well as help you to acquire a cycle buddy or buddies. It can also reinforce your cycling passion to bond with likeminded people.

TIP 2 – A focused effort on consistent cadence on any ride, long or small, group or single, road or hill, is the key in covering distance and getting the best workout.

TIP 3 – To make a group long-distance ride seem less daunting, do this trick: Locate an object or landmark, such as a traffic light or hill, that is off in the distance of your current route. Now intentionally ride to it. Let it pull you to it. After you reach it, find another object or landmark and ride to it too. Do this till you reach your final destination. Setting your aim on a visual object off in the distance, and making a single-minded effort to get to it, will make you unaware of the vast distance that is presently being covered. As a result, miles will pass quickly and effortlessly.

NOTE: Remember, good cycle buddies are hard to find. So, get them where you can. And enjoy the ones you have!

STRANGE ROAD HAZARDS

Modern day riding can present a rider with an array of strange and dangerous hazards to keep an eye out for. As if traffic, weather, and street conditions are not enough.

Given the increase of homelessness and drug use, the streets are more and more becoming the tossing ground to an assortment of bio-waste, drug paraphernalia and the likes. Even nicely paved commuter trails are not exempt from the disgusting things that can litter a path. A rider might come across dog poop, vomit, urine, blood, used condoms, used syringes, and bags of human waste. Sometimes not in a bag. Also, transients throw-away trash in the middle of the trail. All these are not just gross, but are potentially dangerous, if contact is made with them. So, be very careful to avoid them. These dangerous items only add to the usual riding perils of the occasional flat cat, bird, possum or skunk (road pizza), among other things you must ride around on any given street on any given day. But I have to say, it is far better to be on a bike having to navigate around them, than to be on foot, running or jogging.

Another thing to watch for is city weed spraying. They do this every so often for weed abatement. The weed killer is yellow in color. This coloring (probably a dye additive) is most likely used so gardeners or city workers can identify areas already sprayed. You can see where the spraying has occurred by the yellow stain on the pathways. Steer clear, especially if wet. Better safe than sorry.

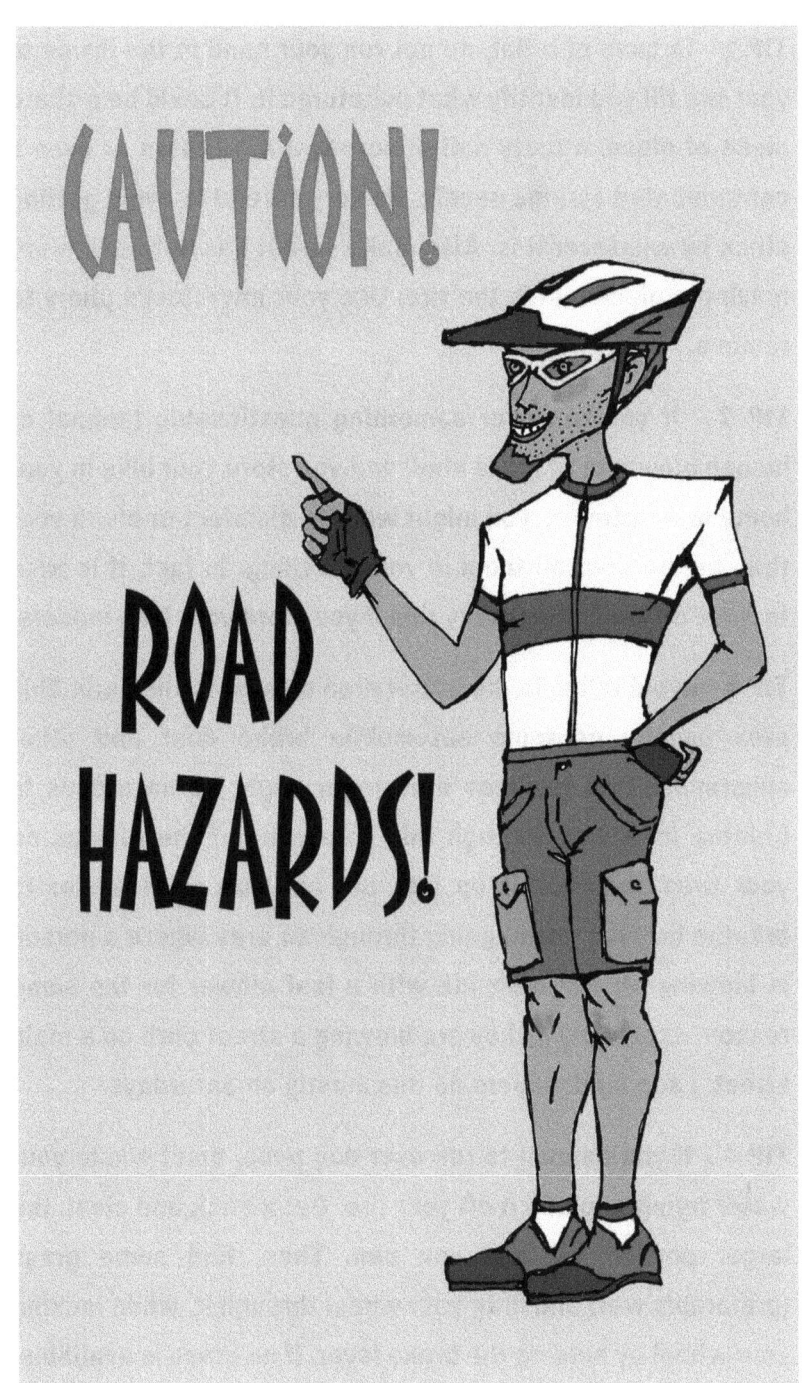

TIP 1 – In case of a flat, do not run your hand in the inside of your tire till you identify what punctured it. It could be a sharp piece of glass, a rusty nail or screw, a dirty thorn or even a contaminated syringe needle. Be very careful to avoid getting stuck by whatever it is. Also make sure it has not broken off, leaving a piece inside the tire. Use your microtool's pliers to remove.

TIP 2 – If you run over something questionable (animal or human biowaste of some kind) and you store your bike in your home or apartment, you might want to disinfect or clean your tires before you roll them in your dwelling. In fact, it is wise to rinse off tires after every ride if you store your bike indoors.

TIP 3 – Avoid riding in the gutter area closest to the curb. This area usually contains automobile brake dust and other substances and residues that are/or might be hazardous to breathe in. Riding through this area will get the residue on your tires and kick it up into the air, making it easier to breathe in. Also, avoid going through an area where a person is blowing off the curbside with a leaf blower for the same reason, especially if they are blowing a street curb on a main street. I see landscapers do this mostly on Saturdays.

TIP 4 – If you happen to run over dog poop, don't waste your water trying to clean it off your tire. Get a stick and clean the larger portion as best you can. Then, find some grass (preferably wet) and drag your wheel through it, while locking your wheel by holding the brake lever. If no grass is available, run your tire through sandy dirt. The dirt will stick to the

mess, and most of it will likely fall off by the time you get home.

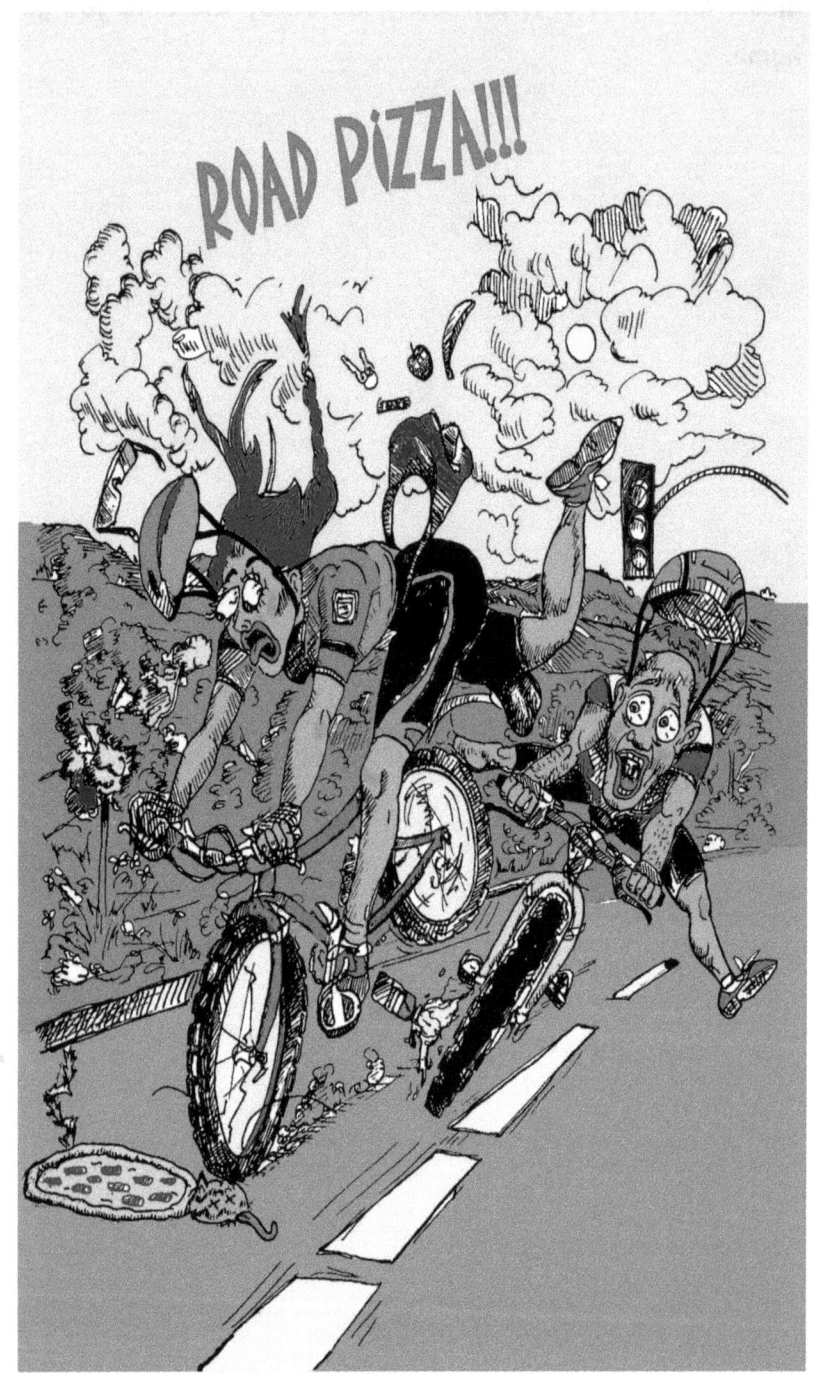

PROTOCOL AND HYGIENE

BE COURTEOUS

Riders just want to have an enjoyable time of cycling on a beautiful day. So, being courteous makes everyone's ride a great ride, and a great ride is a happy ride. Road courtesy is a must and is absolutely free to bestow. One good deed of politeness will beget another, and so on. So be observant and well-intentioned to fellow cyclists, hikers, joggers, and people in cars. Offer gestures of civility where you can. Be a positive force on the road and in the world!

CUSTOMARY SALUTATION

Cyclists are usually friendly with other cyclists. It is the brotherhood/sisterhood of those who share the love for two wheels and freedom. Cycling is a true freedom, the ability to move about covering large distances with relative ease, just using human power. That's something to be excited about! Due to this excitement, cyclists share a great enthusiasm for the ride and usually greet another cyclist with a "hello," "hi," or a nod of the head while passing. Don't feel strange if other cyclists keep greeting you as they pass. Join the brotherhood/sisterhood. Say, "Good morning."

PASSING

Let another rider know if you are going to pass him/her up. This is cycling etiquette and a rule of the road. And when passing another rider, pass on his/her left side.

Common sense and observation tell you that some cyclists veer slightly from side to side or can make abrupt turns as they ride. As a result, a collision can occur if another cyclist is passing that cyclist. A cyclist does not have eyes in the back of his/her head (at least the ones from earth) to see you coming. Most don't ride with a mirror. So, if you need to pass another cyclist, let your presence and intentions be known. Ring your bell, if you have one. However, you must vocalize, "on your left." Remember, the closer you are to the rider you're passing, the slower you need to go. Avoid a collision!

TAILGATING (AKA, WHEEL SUCKING)

"Drafting" can be beneficial if you are riding with a friend or friends. That's when a rider rides closely behind another. The first cyclist breaks the air and rides against it, while the tailing rider benefits by riding easily with no resistance. Energy is saved by the second rider. This was, and still is, mostly done in team racing as riders take turns.

Back in the day, they used to call it "wheel sucking," and it was considered a negative, because the "wheel sucker" was mostly a competing rider stealing a free ride at the energy expense of a rival rider. This is still done today. Not really cool!

In normal riding, alternating positions can be a good cycling strategy between friends on a long ride. But "wheel sucking" on someone you do not know is rude and creepy anywhere.

RIGHT-OF-WAY (WILDERNESS TRAILS)

Here is some basic trail right-of-way etiquette. Trail etiquette can change depending on the trail and state. Also, in the trail designation. So check your park, city, and state rules.

- **Mountain bikers should yield to hikers.**
- **Mountain bikers should yield to equestrian. Mountain biker must pull over to the side of the trail 30ft before the oncoming horse and rider, and dismount till the horse and rider have sufficiently passed.**
- **Mountain bikers traveling downhill should yield to riders heading uphill unless the trail is designated downhill only or one-way.**
- **Motorized vehicles (ATV) must yield to both mountain bikers and hikers, as well as equestrian.**

WISDOM

- If in doubt, assume the hiker has the right-of-way.
- Use a bell when you go around a blind corner.
- Use courtesy, friendliness, and common sense on the trail.

HYGIENE

A TOUCHY SUBJECT (IT MAY BE YOUR BUTT, NOT YOUR SADDLE!)

Sometimes a male rider (maybe female?) may have a sore bum while riding and after, and the saddle is usually blamed. The action of pedaling while sitting has a hair-pulling effect if the rider has neglected the trimming of hair on the buttocks. Simply put, if your bum looks like a bird's nest or nature gone wild, it's time to take a trimmer to it. That is, if you want a pain-free ride. Bum hair can also cause some irritation. Do yourself a favor, or your butt one, and mow the rear yard.

TO SHAVE OR NOT TO SHAVE? (THAT IS THE QUESTION)

It used to be said that shaving the legs (for male cyclists) makes you faster. Maybe, if you are a professional cyclist and are doing a race where every second counts. I do think that it has a psychological boost of making a person feel faster, therefore making a person actually ride faster. It's all about aesthetics, in my opinion.

A male weightlifter will shave for their sport, to make their muscles more pronounced, thus looking more buffed. Same goes for the cyclist. It makes him feel more muscular and anatomical in spandex. It also gives a clean appearance and sporty aerodynamic feel. Plus, it makes it much easier to apply sunblock or lotions and massage sore legs.

Remember that shaving causes tiny micro cuts that are not visible. And given the fact that bike wheels kick up whatever is on the road, like dirty bacteria laden curb water and the likes, one can easily see that tiny cuts provide opportunities for infection. I think that it is far wiser to use an electric trimmer than shaver, since a trimmer causes few cuts, if any. There are also hand-powered hair trimmers that work as well, as an alternative to electric. Nevertheless, as a precaution to either, it's wise to wait a few days after trimming, giving time for any seen or unseen cuts to heal. To the defense of leg hair, I would say that it does provide a barrier (be it ever so slight) to protecting legs from scuff abrasions caused by a tire spinning against a leg.

GENERAL RULE: Do not ride your bike with any open cuts on your body, especially on the legs, even covered with a bandage. There are many life-threatening, easily acquirable bacterial infections a cyclist can get, and spraying tires and road contact with biohazards are the primary source, as I've said. And there is no guarantee that covering a cut with a bandage will keep it 100% safe. Sweat can easily cause a bandage to slip off. Bacteria are small and find their way into a cut. This is the reality of the world in which we live. Dangerous! So, have patience. Yes, it is a big drag to have to wait till any cut or scrape heals to get on the road. But, in this case, the stakes are too high to give in to one's impatience. Best to ride with peace of mind. Wait!

TIP – If I am unsure whether I have open skin on my leg, I simply rub some alcohol on it. Alcohol will burn when it contacts open skin. So it is reasonable to assume this is a good indicator to detect open skin, though, likely not 100% accurate. This works for me.

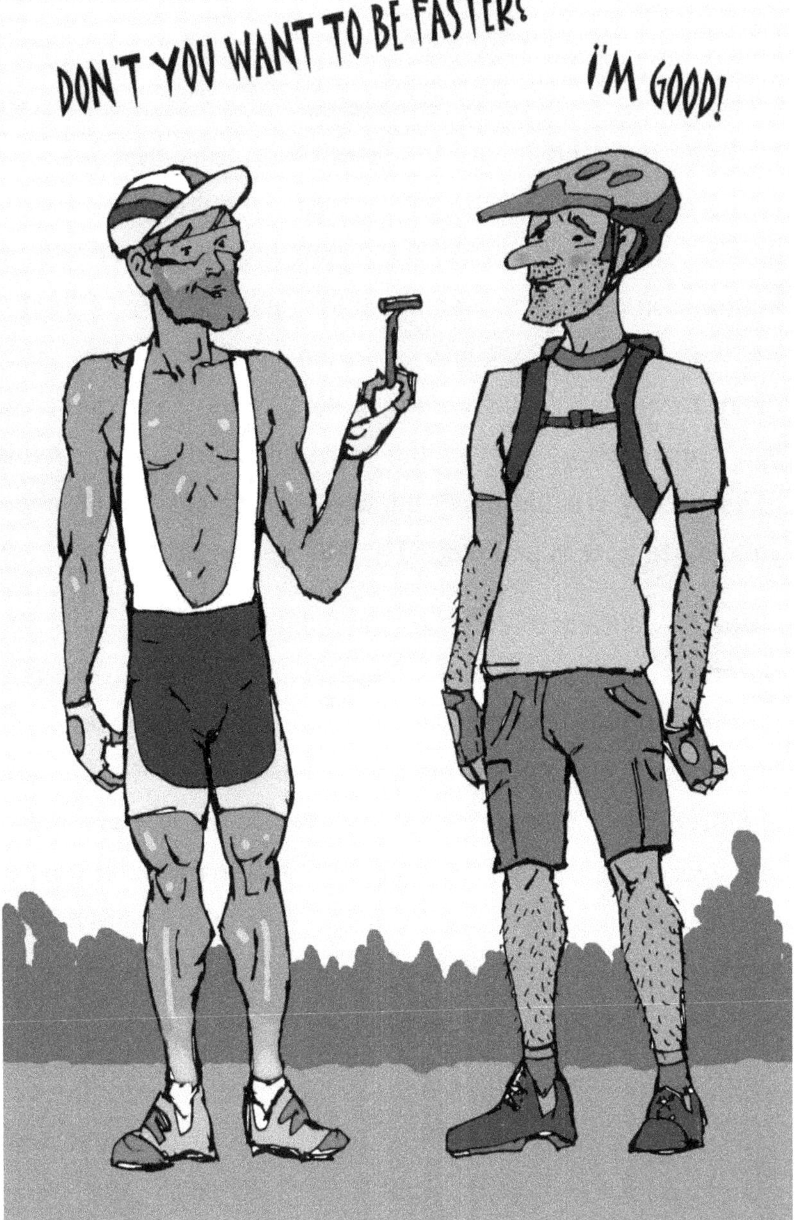
DON'T YOU WANT TO BE FASTER?
I'M GOOD!

MASTER THE ROAD

The road has many obstacles, obstructions, terrain differences, roadkill and forms of difficulties that must be navigated, including near misses and jerks. You must be the master of adaptation and flow. Your goal is to get to your destination with the least amount of resistance and setbacks. So, it is foolish to get into a heated confrontation or react every time a driver has come too close to you or almost hits you. Reckon it as part of the territory and let it go. Avoid unnecessary ordeals. Don't engage everything! Rather, allow yourself to flow in and around and be untouched!

Besides, a great many drivers are just busy, or clueless, and never even noticed you to begin with. I'm not making excuses for them. Again, just let it go! This advice is also relevant to life in general. That being said, all situations are different, and each require a different response. Yes, cyclists have rights like everybody else on the road, but we are at the bottom of the food chain, so to speak, when it comes to our relative size. As in life, choose your fights carefully, but be elusive as far as them finding you.

Another thing, understand the capabilities of your bike and especially your tire and wheel limitations. A thin road bike wheel and tire cannot do what a thick mountain bike wheel and tire can do. So, don't hop curbs or go over questionable things on the road with thin tires. Take care of your bike! With that in mind, look for the path with the least obstacles. Mountain bike downhill riders instinctively eyeball and scan for the smoothest path in the trail, when descending. They do this quickly and automatically. This was especially true and necessary back in the day when mountain bikes had no shocks. But it is fully applicable to any littered path. Scan the road ahead and flow around any obstacles rather than through them. Engage the obstacle only when you have to.

Debris avoidance needs to be observed. Even a small rock in the street can turn into a projectile if your high-pressure tire hits it just right. It can shoot at a parked car 30 feet away, possibly causing paint damage to it. It can also throw off your balance or cause you to crash. There are glass shards, slimy puddles, railroad tracks, gutters, gravel, grates, areas of uneven road, and oil spots that should be **STEERED CLEAR OF**. After a while, avoiding these will become second nature. The adaptable and fluid rider is the best rider. "Be Road Smart!"

NOTE: The absolute best times to bike ride are on holidays like Thanksgiving, Christmas, and New Year's morning. The streets are empty and sweet silence prevails. But keep an eye out for drunk drivers.

NATURE CALLS

This is as good a place as any to mention this. Remember to use the restroom before any extended or small trip, whether a trip on a road or trail.

First, a cyclist normally does not carry a lock for his bike when he or she is riding for sport. A lock and cable are just too heavy and inconvenient. And sport cyclists don't plan to make a stop anyway. So, this creates a bike security problem if you must use a restroom. You can't just leave your bike unattended as you go into a restroom at a stop. What do you do to secure your bike?

Second, finding a restroom can be tough! Where can I go? The search begins in a cold sweat! Restrooms are far and few between in a city. And if you are on the trail, you've got a problem, especially if it's a crowded trail and there is not a bush in sight. Worse, if you are a dude riding with a new girly friend and those tacos with extra sour cream you ate the day before are about to do a number on you. So much for making a good impression! Be aware and think ahead; this can be quite a predicament. So, go before you ride as a rule. As I mentioned earlier in **HYDRATION PACK: ESSENTIALS,** bring two packs of tissue paper, also known as "mountain money," that are individually wrapped, just in case. Packs can be purchased at dollar stores.

TIP – City parks usually have restrooms that are large and open and will accommodate a person rolling his/her bike in with them. Relief is in sight!

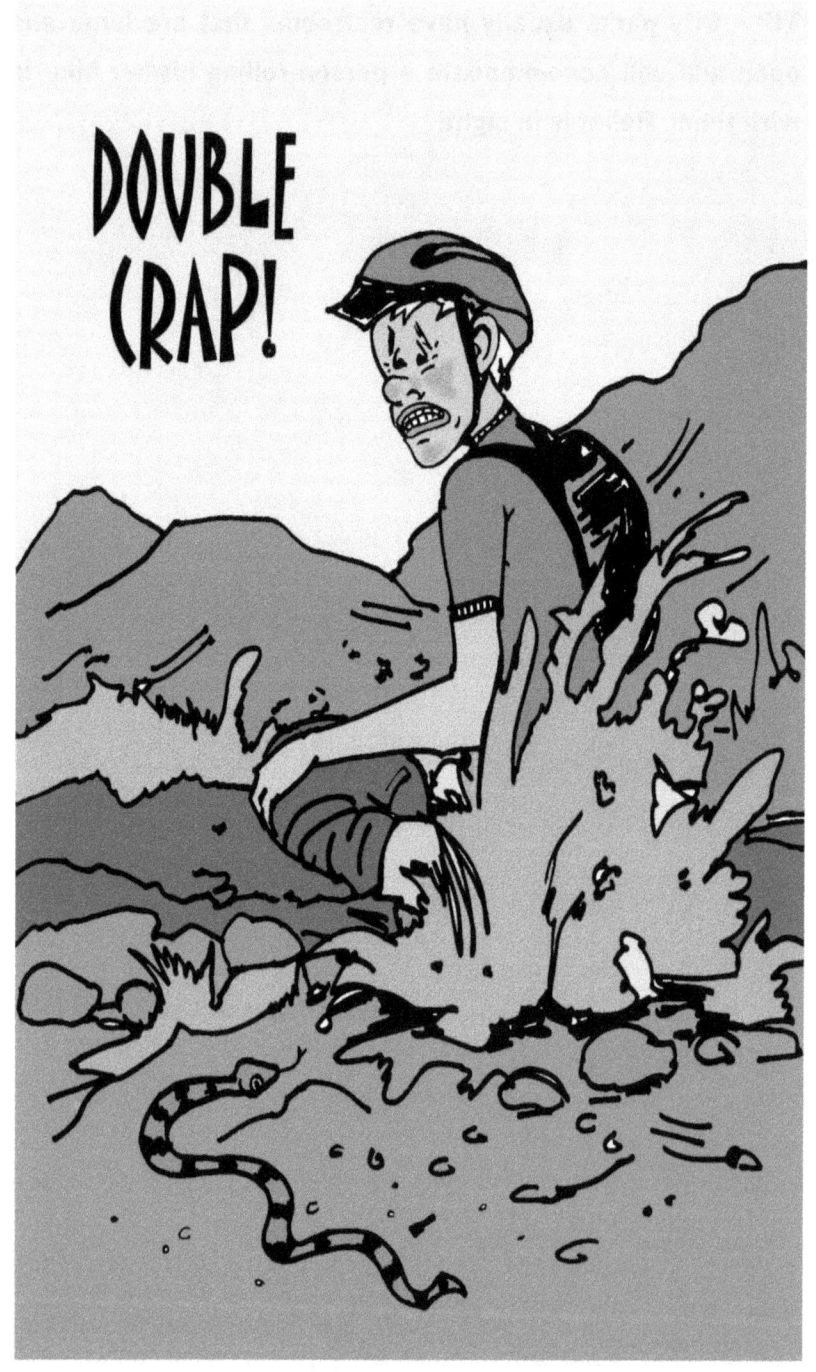

BIKE STORAGE

An important part of owning a bike is deciding where you are going to store it. Some people live in apartments, where there is little or no garage space. Other people live in houses, where they have plenty of garage space. So, it is understandably a question of space that usually dictates the place your bike will be kept. And that might leave your bike in a balcony or small yard.

It is important to understand that your bike should **NEVER** be stored in the open elements for long periods, even with a cover or tarp. The longevity of your bike depends on where and how you store it. The elements destroy a bike in these ways, to name a few:

1) Constant sunlight can fade the finish of your bike, making it look shabby and older than it is.
2) The grips can become ruined after a while; rubber gets sticky and disintegrates. Tires become leathery, lose their bouncy feel, and crack. Seats start to fall apart after a while.
3) Rainwater will get into the frame and cause rust if you have a steel frame. It also gets into the bearings, chain, cables, and shifters, causing them to rust and dry out. The constant hot to cold extremes cause parts to expand

and contract and cause premature aging and cracking on the plastic parts, like shifter casings.

All in all, keeping your bike in the elements is a fast way to destroy your bike. So, keep your bike indoors and be good to it. A bike is a pricey machine!

Remember, even if a bike is in the corner of a room propped against the wall (which is a reasonable place), it can easily fall onto furniture, scratching the furniture or scraping the bike finish. Or even worse, it can fall on a pet. Having a kickstand does not guarantee it will not fall over. These days there are many bike storage devices to keep your bike secure and out of the way while it is not being used. So, take advantage of these, or invent your own hanger—be creative. One advantage to hanging a bike on hooks by the rims or frame is that it prevents flat spots on the tires.

TIP 1 – If you must use a bike cover and you are thrifty (or cheap), you can make a bike cover for about $4.00 by zip tying two 4x6 foot tarps together. Just run to a dollar store (prices can be more than a buck each now) and buy two tarps and a bag of medium zip-ties. Lay one tarp over the other. Now, fold over the edgings (so water can't creep in) and with a pencil poke some holes just under these edgings and push the zip-tie through, and tie. Work your way till you join one 4-foot side and one 6-foot side. Then go only one-third the way down on the last 4-foot side for the front tire opening (See illustration for visuals). You just saved some bucks!

TIP 2 – Speaking about the elements, when washing your bike, avoid spraying water into the wheel bearings. Water can push dirt into the bearings and muck them up. Not good!

TIP 3 – You should buy a plastic storage bin to keep all your bike-related stuff in. Things like extra parts, tubes, patch kits, locks, lights, old grips and whatever. Keep them all in one place and organized.

NOTE: As mentioned earlier, bike accessories are often discounted and put on clearance in department stores, and are a real treasure find. So, buy extras and put them in your bike-stuff bin. Having extras on hand is a great way to be a good friend and help outfit a cycle buddies' bike for little cost to yourself. So, be organized, be stocked, and be a blessing to others!

TARP BIKE COVER

(ROLL & ZIP TIE ALL THE WAY ON ONE 6' AND ONE 4' SIDE)

(AND ONLY 1/3 THE WAY ON THE REMAINING 4' SIDE)

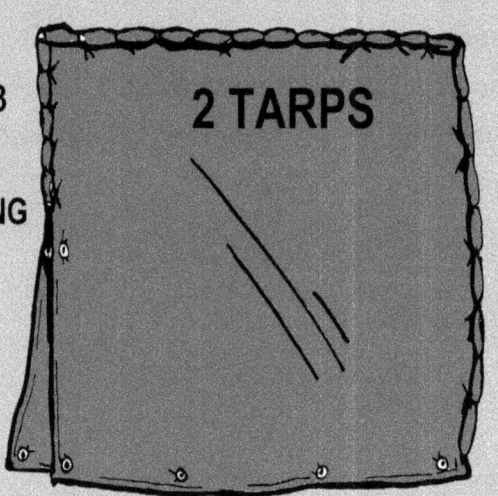

2 TARPS

ONE WITH THE MACHINE

When a rider reaches the point to where he/she no longer just rides a bike, but feels that his/her bike is an extension of his/her person, that rider has now become one with the machine. Not a zen state of so-called enlightenment, but rather a state of fusing with the bike and the ride. By practice, knowledge, and ride wisdom you have arrived. And that is the goal in this book-to help get you there. Because bike riding is one of life's GREAT pleasures!

NOW, GO OUT AND HAVE A GREAT RIDE! BECAUSE NOW AFTER READING AND USING THIS BOOK, YOU HAVE BECOME ...

BIKE SMART!

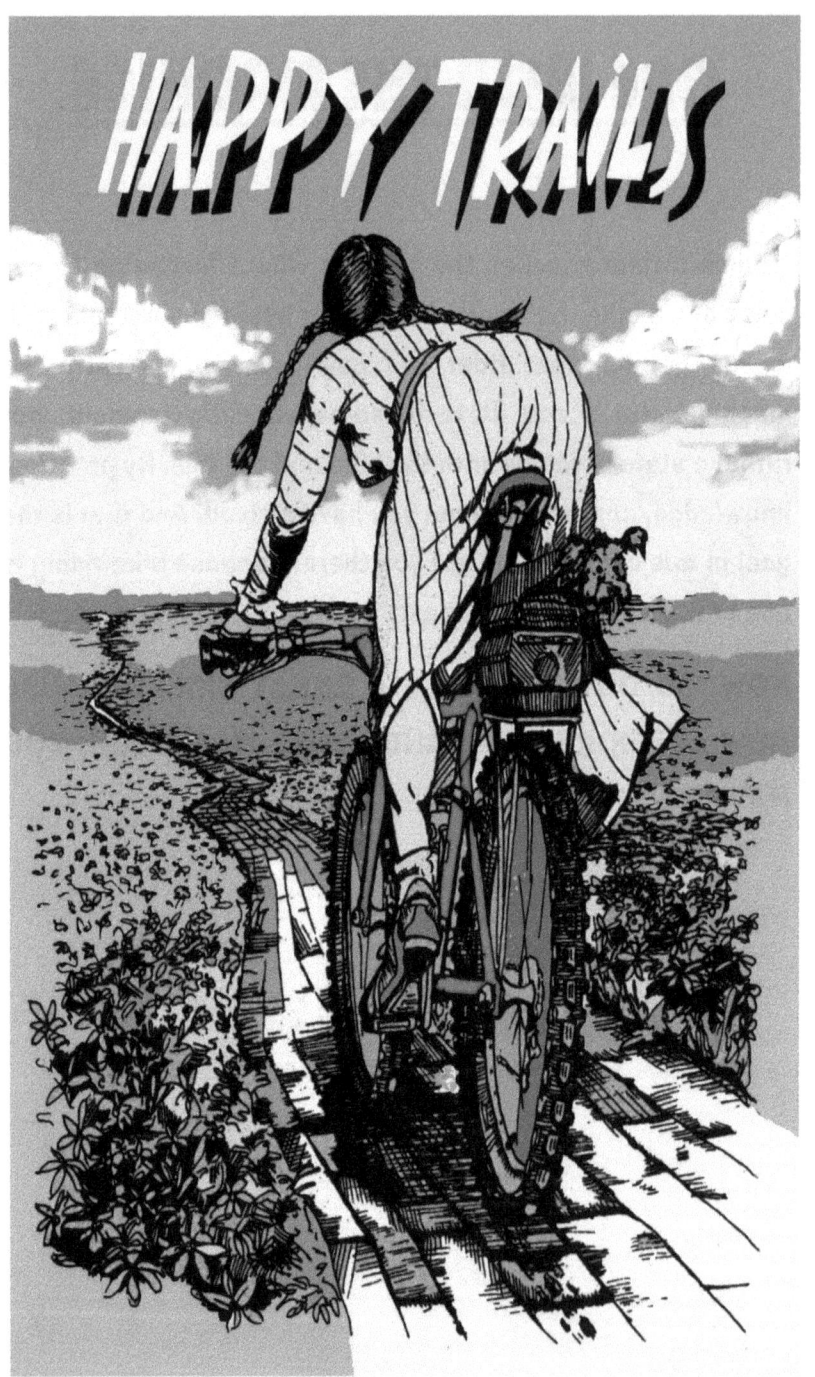

www.ingramcontent.com/pod-product-compliance
Lightning Source LLC
Chambersburg PA
CBHW070138100426
42743CB00013B/2753